**BACTERIOLOGY RESEARCH DEVELOPMENTS**

# *STAPHYLOCOCCUS AUREUS*

# INFECTIONS, TREATMENT AND RISK ASSESSMENT

# BACTERIOLOGY RESEARCH DEVELOPMENTS

Additional books in this series can be found on Nova's website under the Series tab.

Additional e-books in this series can be found on Nova's website under eBook tab.

# IMMUNOLOGY AND IMMUNE SYSTEM DISORDERS

Additional books in this series can be found on Nova's website under the Series tab.

Additional e-books in this series can be found on Nova's website under eBook tab.

BACTERIOLOGY RESEARCH DEVELOPMENTS

# *STAPHYLOCOCCUS AUREUS*

# INFECTIONS, TREATMENT AND RISK ASSESSMENT

MARIA DE LOURDES RIBEIRO
DE SOUZA DA CUNHA
EDITOR

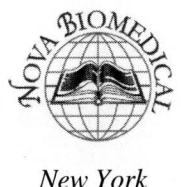

New York

Copyright © 2017 by Nova Science Publishers, Inc.

**All rights reserved.** No part of this book may be reproduced, stored in a retrieval system or transmitted in any form or by any means: electronic, electrostatic, magnetic, tape, mechanical photocopying, recording or otherwise without the written permission of the Publisher.

We have partnered with Copyright Clearance Center to make it easy for you to obtain permissions to reuse content from this publication. Simply navigate to this publication's page on Nova's website and locate the "Get Permission" button below the title description. This button is linked directly to the title's permission page on copyright.com. Alternatively, you can visit copyright.com and search by title, ISBN, or ISSN.

For further questions about using the service on copyright.com, please contact:
Copyright Clearance Center
Phone: +1-(978) 750-8400          Fax: +1-(978) 750-4470          E-mail: info@copyright.com.

## NOTICE TO THE READER

The Publisher has taken reasonable care in the preparation of this book, but makes no expressed or implied warranty of any kind and assumes no responsibility for any errors or omissions. No liability is assumed for incidental or consequential damages in connection with or arising out of information contained in this book. The Publisher shall not be liable for any special, consequential, or exemplary damages resulting, in whole or in part, from the readers' use of, or reliance upon, this material. Any parts of this book based on government reports are so indicated and copyright is claimed for those parts to the extent applicable to compilations of such works.

Independent verification should be sought for any data, advice or recommendations contained in this book. In addition, no responsibility is assumed by the publisher for any injury and/or damage to persons or property arising from any methods, products, instructions, ideas or otherwise contained in this publication.

This publication is designed to provide accurate and authoritative information with regard to the subject matter covered herein. It is sold with the clear understanding that the Publisher is not engaged in rendering legal or any other professional services. If legal or any other expert assistance is required, the services of a competent person should be sought. FROM A DECLARATION OF PARTICIPANTS JOINTLY ADOPTED BY A COMMITTEE OF THE AMERICAN BAR ASSOCIATION AND A COMMITTEE OF PUBLISHERS.

Additional color graphics may be available in the e-book version of this book.

## Library of Congress Cataloging-in-Publication Data

ISBN: 978-1-63485-959-2

Library of Congress Control Number: 2016949776

*Published by Nova Science Publishers, Inc. † New York*

"God, the anchor of our hope"

*I dedicate this book...*
*to my daughters, Taís and Letícia*
*To my parents, Antenor and Alice*

*And especially to the team: Carlos Magno and my students: Aydir, Ana, Camila, Danilo, Lígia, Luiza, Mariana, Natalia, Priscila, Thaís Barbosa and Thaís França who actively participated in the writing of this book.*

# CONTENTS

| | | |
|---|---|---|
| **Preface** | | ix |
| **Chapter 1** | MRSA among Burn Patients: Relevance, Epidemiology and Control<br>*Carlos Magno Castelo Branco Fortaleza and Maria de Lourdes Ribeiro de Souza da Cunha* | 1 |
| **Chapter 2** | Community-Associated *Staphylococcus aureus* (CA-MRSA) in Special Groups<br>*Camila Sena Martins de Souza, Nathalia Bibiana Teixeira and Maria de Lourdes Ribeiro de Souza da Cunha* | 25 |
| **Chapter 3** | Molecular Epidemiology of Livestock-Associated Methicillin-Resistant *Staphylococcus aureus* (LA-MRSA)<br>*Priscila Luiza Mello, Luiza Pinheiro, Lisiane de Almeida Martins and Maria de Lourdes Ribeiro de Souza da Cunha* | 35 |
| **Chapter 4** | Epidemiology of Highly Adaptable Clones: ST398 and Human Diseases<br>*Lígia Maria Abraão, Mariana Fávero Bonesso, Eliane Patrícia Lino Pereira-Franchi and Maria de Lourdes Ribeiro de Souza da Cunha* | 49 |
| **Chapter 5** | *Staphylococcus* spp. in Bloodstream Infections<br>*Aydir Cecília Marinho Monteiro and Maria de Lourdes Ribeiro de Souza da Cunha* | 65 |

| | | |
|---|---|---|
| **Chapter 6** | *Staphylococcus aureus* Infections in Newborns<br>*Danilo Flávio Moraes Riboli, Thaís Alves Barbosa and*<br>*Maria de Lourdes Ribeiro de Souza da Cunha* | **83** |
| **Chapter 7** | *Staphylococcus* spp. in the Etiology of<br>Peritonitis in Peritoneal Dialysis:<br>Risk Factors of the Host and Microorganism<br>*Ana Cláudia Moro Lima dos Santos and*<br>*Maria de Lourdes Ribeiro de Souza da Cunha* | **103** |
| **Chapter 8** | *Staphylococcus aureus*: Superantigens and<br>Autoimmunity<br>*Thais Graziela Donegá França and*<br>*Maria de Lourdes Ribeiro de Souza da Cunha* | **115** |
| **About the Editor** | | **129** |
| **Index** | | **131** |

# PREFACE

This book provides an overview of the different topics of staphylococcal research in recent years. Advances in staphylococcal research are expected on the basis of the information provided for the prediction and prevention of disease.

The epidemiology of *Staphylococcus aureus* and of coagulase-negative staphylococci (CoNS) has undergone a conceptual revolution in recent decades. This phenomenon is due in part to important changes in the epidemiological behavior of these microorganisms. However, there was also reassessment of old concepts in light of new knowledge generated from clinical and experimental research. In this respect, methicillin-resistant *Staphylococcus aureus* (MRSA), which have traditionally been tackled as exclusive agents of healthcare-associated infections, are now recognized as the causative agent of severe disease acquired in the community. In contrast, CoNS have in the past almost been relegated to the role of culture contaminants. This concept was questioned because it contains fundamental lapses: (a) by disregarding the participation of these agents in severe invasive infections; (b) by considering the group to be homogenous in terms of epidemiology and pathogenesis, and (c) by ignoring the role of CoNS as donors of resistance genes for *S. aureus*.

Severe infections caused by bacteria that are resistant to commonly used antibiotics have become a global health problem in the $21^{st}$ century. Since the description of the first MRSA isolates half a century ago, these organisms have spread throughout the world. Although much has been learned about MRSA, we have been completely unable to eradicate them or to consistently prevent the severe infections caused by these microorganisms. MRSA are a threat to global public health because of the rapid propagation and diversification of pandemic clones that are increasingly more virulent and resistant to antimicrobial agents. Furthermore, MRSA are a major cause of healthcare- or hospital-associated infections (HA-MRSA). Burn patients have been indicated as a high-risk group for invasive staphylococcal infection. An important source of *S. aureus* is the burn patient himself if already colonized before the injury. Healthcare workers of the burn unit are another source of colonization. In addition to transmission routes, the clonal nature of *S. aureus* populations also plays an important role. Some strains more successfully colonize the host than others due to the presence of virulence and/or resistance factors that are important for dissemination (Chapter 1).

Antibiotic resistance, which was initially a problem of the hospital environment associated with an increasing number of nosocomial infections that generally affect critically ill and immunodepressed patients, has spread to the community, causing severe illness in previously healthy patients without the traditional vulnerabilities. We now have important organisms that are problematic because of the occurrence of multidrug resistance also in the community. One important example are MRSA, which represent a serious threat to global public health because of the rapid propagation and diversification of pandemic clones that are increasingly more virulent and resistant to antimicrobial agents. Patients infected with community-associated MRSA (CA-MRSA) have not been hospitalized within the past year prior to infection nor had medical procedures such as dialysis, surgery or catheters, facts commonly observed in infections caused by HA-MRSA.

An important aspect of the epidemiology of staphylococci (more specifically *S. aureus*) is the involvement of "special populations". This term should be understood as referring to population strata that differ in terms of ecological pressures and/or specific morbidity conditions. Hence, identification of the prevalence of colonization with *S. aureus* in general, and with MRSA in particular, is of the utmost importance for these populations and may help establish preventive and therapeutic measures for potentially severe infections. As an example, we may cite people living with HIV/AIDS (PLHA). Studies conducted in different countries have shown significant colonization of this population with MRSA, which can be attributed in part to the intense contact with health services. However, MRSA have also been identified in PLHA without a history of hospitalization, invasive procedures, or intravenous medications. This group is characterized by some peculiarities such as the variable degree of immunosuppression and continuous use of medications (notably trimethoprim/sulfamethoxazole), which can interfere with the vulnerability to colonization and infection with HIV. Another particularly vulnerable group are elderly people, who correspond to a growing percentage of the population. In this group, anatomical and physiological factors associated with aging increase the vulnerability to staphylococcal infections, in addition to conditions of mobility and self-care, frequent hospitalizations, and treatment with antibiotics and dressings. Older adults living in long-term care facilities (known as nursing homes) are also submitted to different ecological pressures. Finally, it is necessary to establish the relevance of *Staphylococcus* spp. for patients with chronic diseases, notably diabetes mellitus. Although diabetic patients are known to be more prone to skin and staphylococcal infections, it continues to be necessary to quantify *S. aureus* load and to establish the relevance of MRSA (Chapter 2).

In 2003, a third epidemiological form of MRSA was recognized, which was called livestock-associated MRSA (LA-MRSA). LA-MRSA have been detected in food-producing animals (pigs, cattle, and chicken). In addition to the established risk through direct contact with food-producing animals, the presence of LA-MRSA in human food products demonstrates a possible additional pathway for the transmission of antimicrobial resistance from livestock to the general human population and not only to those who have direct contact with farm animals (Chapter 3).

We believe that a comprehensive and simultaneous approach to the special populations described above, combining epidemiological strategies and the genetic characterization of staphylococci, can provide valuable information. The evaluation of different groups may bring insights into the genesis and dissemination of MRSA lineages. Nowadays, the use of molecular tools permits to outline genetic characteristics and to assess factors that promote high adaptability of certain strains and the success of their persistence. Among these strains, LA-MRSA belonging to clonal complex (CC) 398 are particularly important. Nosocomial infections caused by strains of CC398 are frequently reported. Although it was believed that LA-MRSA CC398 is not easily transmitted between humans, recent reports of hospital transmission of these strains have demonstrated that their potential of dissemination/infection is much higher than previously thought (Chapter 4).

Confirmation of the presence of microorganisms in blood cultures is one of the most important roles of clinical microbiology laboratories. Blood culture testing - the gold standard for the diagnosis of sepsis - is able to elucidate the etiology of infection and to establish appropriate antibiotic treatment in order to improve the prognosis of septic patients and, consequently, to reduce morbidity and mortality. The rapid and efficient identification of these bacteria is important for routine clinical microbiology laboratories. Although automated methods used in routine clinical laboratories are faster, they may not permit accurate identification. Further studies on the efficacy of these systems in identifying these microorganisms are needed. Among CoNS species, *S. epidermidis* and *S. haemolyticus* are the agents most commonly associated with bloodstream infections (Chapter 5).

Nosocomial infections manifest more intensely and more frequently in newborns when compared to children or adults. In addition to the different needs of this age group that render them more susceptible to infection, numerous invasive procedures, the use of broad-spectrum antibiotics and an extended length of stay in the neonatal intensive care unit are factors that can lead to hospital-acquired neonatal infections (Chapter 6).

*Staphylococcus* spp. are an important cause of peritonitis in peritoneal dialysis (PD), frequently requiring change of the dialysis technique and causing an important impact on the mortality of PD patients. In general, peritonitis caused by CoNS has a mild clinical course and a high rate of resolution, but recurrence of apparently cured infections is observed. *Staphylococcus aureus* is associated with more severe episodes and with a poor overall prognosis when compared to other causes of peritonitis, with a higher risk of hospitalization, catheter removal and death. These patients are more likely to require treatment change (Chapter 7).

Epidemiological and experimental evidence supports the theory that infectious agents such as *S. aureus* and its products, the superantigens, are directly related to the development or exacerbation of autoimmune diseases (Chapter 8).

All chapters have gathered together a talented group of contributors, researchers in the field. The book provides an excellent overview of the different applications of staphylococcal research for clinicians, researchers and students who intend to address these issues, and permits continued high-quality research involving these important pathogens.

In: *Staphylococcus aureus*
Editor: M. L. R. S. Cunha

ISBN: 978-1-63485-959-2
© 2017 Nova Science Publishers, Inc.

*Chapter 1*

# MRSA AMONG BURN PATIENTS: RELEVANCE, EPIDEMIOLOGY AND CONTROL

**Carlos Magno Castelo Branco Fortaleza[1] and Maria de Lourdes Ribeiro de Souza da Cunha[2,*]**

[1]Department of Tropical Diseases, Botucatu School of Medicine, Unesp – Univ Estadual Paulista, Botucatu, São Paulo State, Brazil
[2]Department of Microbiology and Immunology, Botucatu Institute of Biosciences, Unesp – Univ Estadual Paulista. Botucatu, São Paulo State, Brazil

## ABSTRACT

Burn wounds provide ideal conditions for colonization and infection with several bacteria. This, alongside with the extensive use of antimicrobials in burn units, facilitates the spread of multidrug-resistant organisms (MDROs). Methicillin-resistant *Staphylococcus aureus* (MRSA) stands out as one of the most threatening MDROs. The burn wound site, degree and extension are associated with greater risk for the acquisition of MRSA. Other factors, such as invasive procedures, prolonged hospitalization and antimicrobial therapy have been associated with MRSA colonization or infection. MRSA-infected patients are at greater risk of death, and may transmit the pathogen to others. The

---

[*] Corresponding author: cunhamlr@ibb.unesp.br

recognition of the clinical importance of MRSA in burn patients highlights the need of appropriate infection control measures that aim to minimize transmission among vulnerable patients. In that setting, the ever changing epidemiology of this microorganism makes it necessary to apply molecular epidemiology methods, in order to identify the circulation of specific clones, the spread of resistance phenotypes and the virulence of strains. Active surveillance of MRSA colonization and infection is an essential part of any strategy aimed at preventing or controlling that agent. In this chapter we will discuss aspects of MRSA epidemiology, antimicrobial resistance and virulence, and their implications for burn patients. We will also address the current recommendations for surveillance and control of MRSA among that population.

## INTRODUCTION

Burn injuries provide the ideal conditions for the colonization, infection and transmission of pathogens and are a frequent cause of morbidity and mortality. The location and extent of burns, invasive procedures, prolonged hospital stay, and antibiotic therapy are risk factors for the colonization with methicillin-resistant *Staphylococcus aureus* (MRSA).

Since the description of the first MRSA isolates half a century ago, these organisms have spread throughout the world. Although much has been learned about MRSA, we have been totally unable to eradicate them or to consistently prevent the severe infections caused by these microorganisms. MRSA are a global threat to public health due to the rapid propagation and diversification of pandemic clones that are increasingly more virulent and resistant to antimicrobial agents. MRSA are a major cause of healthcare or hospital-associated (HA-MRSA) infections. However, the prevalence of infections acquired in the community (community-associated methicillin-resistant *S. aureus*, CA-MRSA) has increased in the last few years. Patients infected with CA-MRSA were not hospitalized in the year prior to infection nor were they submitted to medical procedures such as dialysis, surgery or catheters, facts that are common in nosocomial MRSA infection (HA-MRSA). Whereas HA-MRSA are characterized by broad resistance to different antibiotics, CA-MRSA strains are sensitive (85% to 100%) to drugs such as clindamycin, gentamicin, ciprofloxacin, sulfamethoxazole/trimethoprim and vancomycin, and are only resistant to oxacillin and other beta-lactams [1].

Oxacillin resistance in *S. aureus* is mediated by the production of a supplemental penicillin-binding protein (PBP 2' or PBP 2a), which shows low affinity for semi-synthetic penicillins and is encoded by the *mecA* gene. This gene is carried by a mobile genetic element identified as staphylococcal chromosome cassette *mec* (SCC*mec*) integrated in the chromosome, which comprises the *mec* gene complex, *ccr* gene complex, and region J. The *mec* gene complex consists of the *mecA* gene and its regulatory genes, *mecI* and *mecRI*. The *ccr* gene complex is responsible for the integration and excision of SCC*mec* in the chromosome. In contrast, region J is not essential for the cassette chromosome, but can carry genes encoding resistance to non-beta-lactam antibiotics and heavy metals [2]. The type of SCC*mec* is defined by the combination of the type of the *ccr* gene complex and the class of the *mec* gene complex. SCC*mec* types I-III are found in HA-MRSA, are relatively large, and transport multiple antibiotic resistance determinants. In contrast, SCC*mec* types IV and V are short, do not carry other antibiotic resistance genes, and are found in CA-MRSA [3].

Nasal and pharyngeal colonization of patients, as well as of healthcare workers, seems to play an important role in the dissemination of MRSA. This problem is aggravated in burn patients in whom the normal physical barrier of intact skin is absent. In burn injuries, molecules such as fibronectin, fibrinogen, collagen and many others are exposed on the wound surface [4]. *S. aureus* presents various proteins that specifically interact with human extracellular matrix components, called microbial surface components recognizing adhesive matrix molecules (MSCRAMMs), and permit persistent colonization.

An important source of *S. aureus* is the burn patient himself if already colonized before the injury. In this case, colonization is classified as endogenous. Healthcare workers of the burn unit are another source of colonization. Patients who do not harbor *S. aureus* at the time of admission are prone to become colonized with staphylococci through contact with caregivers. In these cases, colonization can be classified as exogenous or cross-contamination. In addition to transmission routes, the clonal nature of the *S. aureus* populations also plays an important role. Some strains more successfully colonize the host than others due to the presence of virulence and/or resistance factors that are important for dissemination. These strains can cause serious infections.

The understanding of the epidemiology of MRSA infections has important implications for the establishment of control measures. It is therefore necessary to document the dissemination of MRSA clones and to identify individual factors related to their acquisition. More virulent MRSA clones are emerging both in hospitals and in the community and there is evidence that virulence factors can be transferred between nosocomial and community-associated clones by recombination. Clinicians should be aware of the variable antimicrobial resistance profile of MRSA clones circulating in the region in order to select the most appropriate empirical antibiotic therapy. In this respect, regional epidemiology programs need to be established for the precise identification and characterization of circulating MRSA clones.

Surveillance systems that monitor the dissemination of MRSA, antibiotic resistance profile, virulence of strains and risk factors associated with infection are essential so that preventive and therapeutic measures of MRSA infection are used effectively. The objective of this chapter is to discuss aspects related to the epidemiology of MRSA, antibiotic resistance, virulence, MRSA surveillance, and infection control strategies in burn patients.

## *STAPHYLOCOCCUS AUREUS*: MORPHOLOGY, PATHOGENESIS, RESISTANCE

The genus *Staphylococcus* comprises different species and subspecies, which are widely distributed in nature and are mainly found on the skin and mucous membranes of birds and mammals [5]. Staphylococci are immobile, facultative anaerobic, mesophilic, non-sporulating, and catalase-positive Gram-positive bacteria. Fifty-two species and 28 subspecies have so far been described for the genus [6], most of them coagulase-negative. *Staphylococcus aureus* has always been the most important species and has been associated with a series of infections in humans and animals. Several virulence factors are responsible for the symptoms and severity of community- and hospital-acquired infections caused by *S. aureus*, which are currently a leading clinical and epidemiological problem in healthcare-associated infections. These microorganisms are important because of their pathogenicity and high frequency, causing diseases in both immunocompromised and healthy individuals due to their easy intrahospital dissemination and enormous capacity of adaptation and antibiotic resistance [7].

The arsenal of virulence factors of *S. aureus* is extensive. Some of these factors are part of the structure of the cell itself and others are extracellular factors that are produced during growth and eliminated into the extracellular medium. Both types of factors play an important role in the pathogenesis of infection. *S. aureus* expresses dozens of proteins found on the bacterial surface, called microbial surface components recognizing adhesive matrix molecules (MSCRAMMs), including collagen-binding protein, fibronectin-binding protein, elastin-binding protein, and fibrinogen-binding protein, which bind specifically to extracellular matrix proteins of the host, thus permitting adherence to host tissue. These proteins seem to play a key role in the onset of staphylococcal infections. After adhering to host tissues, catheters or prostheses, *S. aureus* is able to grow and persist by forming a biofilm that permits evasion of the host immune response and antimicrobial action. The ability of biofilm formation is one of the reasons that catheter- or prosthesis-associated infections are difficult to eradicate without removal of the device [8].

*S. aureus* possesses other characteristics that help evade the host immune system during infection. A polysaccharide capsule is produced by approximately 90% of clinical isolates, and two serotypes, capsule types 5 and 8, are found in 75% of *S. aureus* isolated from humans. The main virulence function of the capsule is to prevent phagocytosis, but it has also been associated with the colonization and persistence of *S. aureus* on mucous membranes [9]. Protein A is also part of the cell wall and binds to fraction Fc of immunoglobulins, preventing opsonization [10].

In contrast to protective and passive virulence factors associated with the cell wall during infection, *S. aureus* produces numerous extracellular enzymes such as proteases and lipases that permit the microorganism to invade and destroy the host tissue and to spread to other sites. In addition to these enzymes, various toxins are released into the extracellular medium, including superantigens and cytolytic toxins. More than 20 different superantigens have been identified, including staphylococcal enterotoxins (SEs), staphylococcal enterotoxin-like (SEl) toxins, toxic shock syndrome toxin 1 (TSST-1), and exfoliative toxins (ETs). Superantigens have the ability to stimulate and activate T lymphocytes, inducing the production of high levels of cytokines that cause the symptoms observed in toxic shock syndrome, as well as anergy, inflammation, cytotoxicity, T cell deletion and autoimmunity [11, 12], thus facilitating colonization of the individual.

Cytolytic toxins also play an important role in the development of staphylococcal infections. These toxins include $\alpha$-toxin, $\beta$-toxin, $\delta$-toxin, $\gamma$-toxin, Panton-Valentine leukocidin (PVL), and phenol-soluble modulin (PSM), which destroy leukocytes by forming pores in the cell membrane, causing tissue necrosis and permitting escape from the host immune system. Alpha-toxin is the best-characterized toxin, which is encoded by the *hla* gene and carried by almost all clinical isolates of *S. aureus*. This toxin has a broad spectrum of activity against a wide range of cells, including erythrocytes, leukocytes (monocytes, macrophages and polymorphonuclear cells [PMNs]), platelets, epithelial cells, and fibroblasts, exerting hemolytic, dermonecrotic and neurotoxic activity. In addition, the toxin is lethal when injected intravenously and necrotizing activity associated with pneumonia has been demonstrated in a murine model [13]. Beta-toxin is a sphingomyelinase C. As a consequence, the sensitivity of human cells to this toxin depends on the amount of sphingomyelin in the membrane. Beta-toxin is cytotoxic to monocytes, erythrocytes, neutrophils and lymphocytes. Recently, this toxin has been reported to play a role in the production of a nucleoprotein matrix during staphylococcal biofilm formation. Gamma-toxin and PVL consist of two protein components, called slow (S)-eluting and fast (F)-eluting. Gamma-toxin containing the S (HlgA or HlgC) and F (HlgB) components causes lysis of leukocytes and erythrocytes, whereas PVL (formed by lukS-PV and lukF-PV) is toxic to leukocytes [14]. PVL is associated with extensive tissue necrosis and is responsible for severe skin infections and necrotizing pneumonia.

The *lukS-PV* and *lukF-PV* genes that encode PVL are carried by a specific bacteriophage (*phiSLT*) that infects and lyses *S. aureus* cells, integrating the PVL genes into the chromosome of this microorganism. Once the LukS-PV and LukF-PV proteins are transcribed and secreted, they form a heptamer that causes cell lysis of PMNs. Depending on the concentration of the toxin, PMNs undergo lysis or apoptosis. In view of these facts, the action of PVL may not be directly related to tissue necrosis, but rather to the release of cytotoxic lysosomal granules during PMN lysis, to reactive oxygen released from granulocytes, or even to the inflammatory cascade [15]. Delta-toxin is a 26-amino acid peptide that is cytolytic to human erythrocytes, neutrophils, and other mammalian cells. It is believed that the toxin acts as a surfactant, disrupting cellular membranes. This toxin is produced by 97% of *S. aureus* isolates. Wang et al. [16] suggested that this toxin is structurally similar to the so-called phenol-soluble modulins (PSMs), a family of peptides with hemolytic and proinflammatory activity. The authors showed that CA-MRSA isolates produced high amounts of PSMs (including δ-toxin), and strains in which the PSM genes were deleted were less virulent in experimental models of skin infection and bacteremia in rats. *S. aureus* also produces PSMs, which are carried by mobile genetic elements such as SCC*mec*, thus combining resistance and virulence on the same genetic element.

At present, resistance of *Staphylococcus* to methicillin is a global health problem and studies conducted throughout Europe, America, Asia and Africa have demonstrated the predominance of MRSA over methicillin-susceptible isolates. In Europe, the prevalence of MRSA ranges from 1% in countries such as Norway and The Netherlands to rates higher than 50% in Spain, Italy and Portugal [17]. In the United States, the prevalence of MRSA was 55.2% in 2007/2008 and 54.6% in 2009/2010, with a 1.7% reduction in the percentage of resistance, but the difference was not significant [18]. In Brazil, the estimated frequency of oxacillin resistance is high among *S. aureus* strains, especially those isolated from large medical centers and university hospitals. Studies conducted at the Hospital of the Botucatu School of Medicine (Hospital da Faculdade de Medicina de Botucatu), São Paulo, reported rates of 18% for the neonatal and pediatric ICUs and of 50% for adult wards and ICU [19, 20]. Chen et al. [21] found an overall prevalence of MRSA of 55.3% at four burn centers in China, with the rates ranging from 36.7% to 86.4% at the four centers studied.

Oxacillin resistance in *S. aureus* is mediated by the production of a supplemental penicillin-binding protein (PBP 2' or PBP 2a), which shows low affinity for semi-synthetic penicillins. This protein is encoded by the chromosomal *mecA* gene. Whereas staphylococcal strains normally employ three PBPs (1, 2 and 3) for cell wall synthesis, MRSA possess one supplemental PBP (PBP 2' or PBP 2a). Therefore, when the *mecA* gene is present, the cell is able to grow in the presence of oxacillin and other beta-lactams.

The *mecA* gene is carried by a mobile genetic element identified as staphylococcal cassette chromosome *mec* (SCC*mec*), which is integrated into a specific site of the chromosome, called *orfx*, and comprises the *mec* gene complex, *ccr* gene complex and region J. The *mec* gene complex consists of the *mecA* gene and its regulatory genes *mecI* and *mecRI*. The *ccr* gene complex is responsible for the integration and excision of SCC*mec* in the chromosome. In contrast, region J is not essential for the cassette chromosome, but can carry genes encoding resistance to non-beta-lactam antibiotics and heavy metals [2]. Eleven types of SCC*mec* have been described so far, which are defined by the combination of the type of the *ccr* gene complex and the class of the *mec* gene complex. Subtypes are defined by polymorphisms in region J in the same combination of *mec* and *ccr* complexes [2].

SCC*mec* typing is a useful epidemiological tool [22] since different types are more prevalent in the hospital or community setting. The prevalence of infections caused by CA-MRSA, including skin and soft tissue infections, has been increasing worldwide since the 1990s. This increased frequency and consequent morbidity and mortality associated with infections caused by these microorganisms indicate that these infections could become a public health problem. SCC*mec* types I, II and III are found in most hospital isolates. Community-acquired MRSA strains usually carry SCC*mec* type IV and, less frequently, type V. Although SCC*mec* type IV is associated mainly with CA-MRSA, a pediatric MRSA clone, called USA 800, exists which causes nosocomial infections and also carries *mecA* on SCC*mec* type IV.

In areas where the levels of infection with MRSA carrying SCC*mec* type IV are high, non-beta-lactam antibiotics, such as sulfamethoxazole-trimethoprim, clindamycin or tetracycline, should be administered since most of these strains are susceptible to these drugs. First, these antibiotics should be used for empirical treatment of uncomplicated skin and soft tissue infections. Changes in antibiotic therapy should be based on the results of antimicrobial susceptibility testing. Vancomycin is recommended for the treatment of infections caused by HA-MRSA, since SCC*mec* type III strains are usually resistant to other beta-lactams, macrolides, aminoglycosides, chloramphenicol, quinolones, and tetracycline [23, 24]. However, in 1996, the first clinical isolate of *S. aureus* with reduced vancomycin susceptibility (intermediate MIC = 8 μg/ml), called vancomycin-intermediate *S. aureus* (VISA), was reported in Japan [25]. Subsequently, reports of vancomycin-resistant *S. aureus* (VRSA) occurred in the United States by 2002. Other more recent classes of antibiotics such as streptogramins (quinupristin/dalfopristin), oxazolidine (linezolid), glycylcycline (tigecycline) and lipopeptides (daptomycin) are available, and other antimicrobials are currently being evaluated, including ceftobiprole, dalbavancin, oritavancin, and televancin.

## EPIDEMIOLOGICAL ASPECTS (HA-MRSA, CA-MRSA)

Molecular epidemiological studies have highlighted the continuous global evolution/propagation of MRSA clones and their increasing antibiotic resistance and virulence. We only have partial understanding of the factors that contribute to the propagation of MRSA clones, but these factors are likely to include the migration of human populations, ineffective methods for the control MRSA transmission by infected patients, and poorly effective treatment strategies including the inadequate use/choice of antibiotics. In hospitals, patients already carrying MRSA at the time of admission are at higher risk of contracting an infection derived from colonizing bacteria or of transmitting MRSA to other patients [26].

The understanding of the epidemiology of MRSA infections has important implications for the establishment of control measures. It is therefore necessary to document the dissemination of MRSA clones and to identify individual factors related to their acquisition. Pulsed-field gel electrophoresis (PFGE) continues to be the most commonly method used in micro-epidemiology studies (local outbreaks). This method is based on the restriction (typically *SmaI*) of bacterial genomic DNA and subsequent separation of the fragments by gel electrophoresis in an alternating electrical field.

Although PFGE is an adequate technique for the study of outbreaks, it is not sufficient for long-term or global epidemiological studies [27]. Studies on the clonality of *S. aureus* are frequently complemented by a technique called multilocus sequence typing (MLST). This method is based on the analysis of seven housekeeping genes of the microorganism, in which different sequences correspond to different alleles of each gene and to a so-called sequence type (ST). The results are deposited in the MLST database at http://www.mlst.net, which permits comparisons between *S. aureus* sequences described in different parts of the world.

Another commonly used typing method is *spa* typing developed by Frenay et al. [28], which determines sequence variation in the polymorphic X-region of the protein A gene of *S. aureus*. In this method, the protein A gene (*spa*) is amplified by PCR and sequenced for detection of the polymorphic X-region or short sequence repeats (SSR). The SSR region of the *spa* gene is subject to spontaneous mutations, as well as the loss or gain of repeats. Alphanumeric codes are attributed to these repeats and the *spa* type is deduced from the order of specific repeats [29]. *Spa* typing has been shown to be useful for both the study of molecular evolution and nosocomial MRSA outbreaks. A universal nomenclature and public access to the *spa* typing data are guaranteed by the SeqNet.org initiative (www.seqnet.org), which synchronizes all *spa* typing data with the central *spa* server (http://spaserver.ridom.de) [30].

The combination of various molecular typing techniques resulted in the identification of five MRSA clones widely disseminated worldwide. These clones, called Iberian, Brazilian/Hungarian, New York/Japan, pediatric and EMRSA-16, account for 68% of all MRSA and are the most successful in terms of the ability to cause infection, persistence, and the capacity of dissemination from one geographic area to another and even in different continents [31]. These clones were named according to the geographic area where they were first described (Brazilian epidemic clone, Iberian clone, New

York/Japan clone), the epidemiological characteristics of the patients from which they were isolated (pediatric clone), PFGE pattern (USA 100, USA 800), or phage type (EMRSA-15, EMRSA-16) [1]. The international nomenclature of MRSA clones is currently based on MLST and SCC*mec*, and almost all MRSA infections in the world are caused by five predominant pandemic clones (ST5-HA-MRSA-II [New York/Japan], ST5-HA-MRSA-IV [pediatric], ST-247-HA-MRSA [Iberian], ST-239-HA-MRSA-III [Brazilian-Hungarian], and ST30-CA-MRSA-IV [Oceania Southwest Pacific clone, OSPC]).

The characterization of these clones is important to formulate adequate local therapeutic strategies. For example, more complete knowledge of the clones circulating in a given region can be used to evaluate the relationship between clonal types, symptoms of the disease, choice of antibiotics, and clinical results. Furthermore, an important and necessary step to develop more effective strategies for the control of MRSA propagation in a given region is to understand why specific clones predominant in different regions.

## BURN WOUND INFECTIONS

The burn wound is characterized by varied areas of necrosis, ischemia and inflammation. This picture is easily confounded with an infection, and – paradoxically – provides an ideal site of entry for microorganisms [32]. Therefore, authors have proposed criteria that can be applicable on the bedside to diagnose a possible infection, and therefore introduce appropriate therapy [33].

*S. aureus*, and MRSA in particular is, alongside with Gram-negative bacilli such as *Pseudomonas aeruginosa* and *Acinetobacter baumannii*, one of the most frequent agents of burn wound infections [32, 34]. The clinical picture is similar for those pathogens, and involves changes in the aspect of the burn wound and extension of the affected areas, often with inflammation of skin and soft tissues that surround the wound. Moreover, symptoms and signs that are common to other infection sites, such as fever, tachycardia and tachypnea are often present [34]. They may be accompanied by elevations in white blood cell counts and inflammatory markers, such as the C-reactive protein [35, 36]. Those parameters may indicate a progression to sepsis. Therefore, criteria have been proposed to diagnose sepsis in this setting. We will discuss them in the next section.

Besides clinical suspicion, the microbiologic diagnosis of burn wound infections is challenging. The "gold standard" for diagnosis is the histological analysis of viable tissue showing microbial invasion [32]. Due to the relatively long time for results and other operational concerns, this technique is rarely used nowadays [37, 38]. Cultures of the skin, either by swabs or biopsy, have poor accuracy and do not discriminate asymptomatic colonization from true infections [39]. Still, some authors argue that quantitative culture of tissue specimens may point out to the most prevalent bacterial agent in the burn wound site, and this information – altogether with the clinical criteria for infection – may help directing therapy [32]. Moreover, there is evidence for a negative predictive value for quantitative cultures yelding less than $10^5$ colony forming units/gram [33]. Despite all controversy, most authors advise a combination of culturing secretions and/or tissues altogether with taking blood cultures and interpreting results in the light of coherence with clinical parameters.

The prevention of burn wound infections typically involves repeated burn wound excisions and topical antimicrobial agents (e.g., silver sulfadiazine). In spite of the widespread performance of both measures, their precise role in infection prevention is unclear [36]. Burn wound excisions and closure are believe to reduce the entry of infectious agents (including MRSA). They have been performed more often in recent times, and may account for the continuous decrease in burn wound infections that is generally reported [40]. Paradoxically, two sequential studies conducted in a burn unit in Brazil associated the number of excisions to the risk of acquiring MRSA [41, 42]. However, results may be confounded, and it is possible that the number of excisions is a proxy of the severity of the burn wound. The use of systemic antimicrobials in prophylaxis is advisable only in perioperative period. However, one systematic review suggested a beneficial effect for continuous prophylaxis with systemic agents [43]. Though promising, this is still an unresolved issue.

## OTHER MRSA INFECTIONS AFFECTING BURN PATIENTS

Burned patients, especially those with severe burns, often require critical care. They are thus submitted to invasive procedures and insertion of several devices. Surgical site infections, central-line related bloodstream infections and ventilator-associated pneumonia are frequent in this group, and MRSA is one of the leading etiologic agents [34, 44].

Surgical procedures provide an additional opportunity for the microbial invasion of body sites. Surgical site infections (SSI) may arise in burn patients in surgeries involving skin (e.g., grafting) or bones and joints (including amputation). Also, burn patients may present multiple visceral trauma and or other complications requiring surgery beyond the burned surface. In all those settings, SSI provides additional morbidity and mortality [44]. Therefore, efforts directed to its prevention (asepsis of the skin, appropriate use of antimicrobial prophylaxis, optimized surgical technique) are of utmost importance. Once the infection is diagnosed – through presence of inflammation and/or pus in the surgical wound or imaging evidence of deep abscesses – therapy must be instituted. When there are foreign bodies related to the procedure, they should ideally be removed – since they may harbour biofilms that hinder the effect of antimicrobials [45].

Ventilator-associated pneumonia (VAP) poses a severe threat for burn patients. According to the 2011 report from the National Healthcare Safety Network (NHSN), the overall incidence for VAP was 4.9 per 1,000 ventilator-days [46]. However, there are reports of rates as high as 26 per 1,000 ventilator-days [47, 48, 49]. Specific risk factors for VAP include inhalation injury, older age, length of admission and/or intubation and the total body surface affected [47, 50]. The diagnosis of VAP is challenging, and relies on medical and laboratorial criteria. The NHSN made several updates to criteria used for surveillance, and since 2013 abandoned those criteria in favour of the more accurate monitoring of "ventilator-associated events" (CDC). Still, for clinical purposes, there remains a definition including new and persistent chest infiltrate, altogether with change in characteristics of the sputum and a sepsis picture (fever, tachycardia, high or low white blood cell counts) [51]. Preventive measures for VAP include elevating the patients head, aseptic manipulation of the respiratory apparatus and oral hygiene – among other recommendations. Still, this infectious syndrome remains the most controversial as regards to the evidence for preventive strategies [52]. However, since the mortality attributed to VAP is high (especially when it involves MDR pathogens such as MRSA), empiric or culture-driven antimicrobials should be promptly instituted for any suspected case [53].

Central line-associated bloodstream infections (CLABSI) manifests clinically as sepsis syndrome without any specific focus – when it is probable that the site of entry of microorganisms is a catheter placed on a central vein [54, 55]. Its diagnosis involves the presence of positive blood cultures - one for typical pathogens such as MRSA, two for usual contaminants (e.g., coagulase-negative Staphylococci). In the burn patient, it is necessary to differentiate this picture from bacteraemias arising from skin infections, especially after surgical manipulation of tissues (e.g., wound excisions). A popular diagnostic strategy involves simultaneous culture of blood samples and of the tip of central line catheter [56]. Preventive measures are based on aseptic technique during catheter insertion and manipulation. Therapeutic strategies usually require the removal of the catheter, although specific cases (especially those involving long-term catheters) may be elegible to "lock therapy". Briefly, lock therapy involves the use of high concentration intraluminal antibiotics in order to destroy the biofilm attached to the catheter. Regardless of the use of this strategy, parenteral antimicrobials (see bellow) must be administered for patients with CLABSI [56].

Of note, patients with urinary catheters are also highly susceptible to urinary tract infections (UTI). Compared to the sites discussed above, UTI have lower severity, and *S. aureus* is rarely involved in its ethiology [57].

## THERAPY

The anti-MRSA arsenal includes glycopeptides, lipopeptides, oxazolidinones and 5th generation cephalosporins [58]. Vancomycin (a glycopeptide) remains the cornerstone for MRSA therapy [59]. This is due to several aspects. First, MRSA are still widely susceptible to this agent. It is true that the emergence of intermediary susceptible and (rarely) resistant stains has been detected [60]. Also, isolates with minimum inhibitory concentrations above 2 have been associated to therapeutic failure. However, those situations are either uncomon (intermediary susceptibility, resistance) or of unproven relevance [61, 62, 63]. A second advantage of vancomycin is the possibility of adjusting dosing strategies based on monitoring of serum concentrations of this antimicrobial [64]. Finally, most newer drugs have proven at best non-inferior to vancomycin in clinical trials and meta-analysis [58].

An exception is Linezolid (an oxazolidinone), which presented superioriority to vancomycin for treating skin infections [65]. While the specific case for burn wound infections is less clear, Linezolid show promise as a therapeutic option. Superiority of Linezolid (as compared to vancomycin) for pneumonia was found in a large trial [66], but not confirmed in recent meta-analysises [67, 68]. An important limitation for Linezolid is its poor performance in bloodstream infections.

Daptomycin is a lipopeptide with good activity for bloodstream and skin infections. In most studies, its results were comparable to those found for vancomycin. However, inactivation by surfactant prevents its use for the therapy of pneumonia [69].

Fifth generation cephalosporins (Ceftaroline, Ceftobiprole) are also promising for MRSA therapy. Both proved non-inferior to vancomycin for therapy of skin infections in serveral trials. More evidence is needed for efficacy in other infectious sites [70, 71]. Other new antimicrobials (Tigecycline, Telavancin, Quinupristin/Dalfopristin) have anti-MRSA activity. However, there are insufficient data about their effectivity for severe infections [72].

Finally, several MRSA isolates (especially those harboring SCCmec types IV or beyond) present variable susceptibility to Thrimethoprim/ Sulfametoxazole, Clyndamycin and fluorquinolones. The usefulness of those agents for the therapy of infections affecting burn patients is unknown, and they should be used with caution [73]

## Infection Control Issues

The control of MRSA in burn units involves several steps. Usual measures for preventing healthcare-associated infections (e.g., VAP, CLABSI, skin and soft tissue infections) are obviously warranted [40]. Hand hygiene must be emphasized in every policy that aims at preventing and controlling MRSA spread [74, 75, 76].

Isolation precautions for contact transmission are recommended for controlling multidrug-resistant pathogens among patients admitted to hospitals [77, 78]. Keeping MRSA harboring subjects under precautions may prevent cross-transmission, either direct or involving fomites. Even though there is controversy in this issue, most authors advise direct screening for MRSA carriage (surveillance cultures) though collection of swabs from nares and burn wounds (and eventually oropharynx, axillae and perineum) [79]. Each and every subject from whom MRSA was isolated from clinical or surveillance cultures should be placed under precautions.

Other infection control measures include chlorexidine bathing [80] and selective digestive decontamination with oral administration of non-absorbable antibiotics [81]. Those strategies show promise, but require more extensive research in this specific setting (i.e., burn units).

## CONCLUSION

Routine surveillance cultures of nasal swabs obtained during admission of the patient for the detection of colonization with *S. aureus* may identify patients who are at higher risk of developing subsequent staphylococcal infection, and the isolation of these patients colonized with MRSA may prevent cross-transmission.

The different MRSA lineages cause variable types of infections, which vary in terms of severity from skin infections to severe sepsis with a life-threatening risk. The severity of disease is usually directly related to the production of specific virulence factors by MRSA, such as toxins or protective biofilms, whereas the propagation of MRSA depends in part on the capacity of each clone to acquire resistance to antibacterial agents.

The use of molecular typing techniques of clinical isolates permits to identify clones that predominate in a unit and may contribute to elucidate the source of MRSA infections so that more effective treatments and more adequate prevention strategies can be planned.

## REFERENCES

[1] Chambers, HF; Deleo, FR. Waves of resistance: *Staphylococcus aureus* in the antibiotic era. *Nat Rev Microbiol.*, 2009,7(9), 629-41.

[2] (IWG-SCC) International Working Group on the Classification of Staphylococcal Cassete Chromosome Elements. Classification of staphylococcal cassette chromosome *mec* (SCC*mec*): guidelines for reporting novel SCC*mec* elements. *Antimicrob Agents Chemother.*, 2009, 53(12), 4961-7.

[3] Ito, T; Katayama, Y; Asada, K; Mori, N; Tsutsumimoto, K; Tiensasitorn, C; et al. Structural comparison of three types of staphylococcal cassette chromosome *mec* integrated in the chromosome in methicillin-resistant *Staphylococcus aureus*. *Antimicrob Agents Chemother.*, 2001, 45(5), 1323-36.

[4] Krivan, HC; Roberts, DD; Ginsburg, V. Many pulmonary pathogenic bacteria bind specifically to the carbohydrate sequence GalNAcβ1–4Gal found in some glycolipids. *Proc Natl Acad Sci USA.*, 1988, 85, 6157-61.

[5] Kloos, WE; Bannerman, TL. *Staphylococcus* and *Micrococcus*. In: Murray PR, Baron EJ, Pfaller MA, Tenover FC, Yolken RH, editors. *Manual of Clinical Microbiology*. Washington: American Society for Microbiology Press, 1999, p. 264-282.

[6] Euzéby, JP. List of prokaryotic names with standing in nomenclature – Genus *Staphylococcus*. Acesso em: 28 jul 2016. Disponível em: http://www.bacterio.cict.fr/s/staphylococcus.html.

[7] Enright, MC; Robinson, DA; Randle, G; Feil, EJ; Grundmann, H; Spratt, BG. The evolutionary history of methicillin-resistant *Staphylococcus aureus* (MRSA). *Proc Natl Acad Sci U S A.*, 2002, 99(11),7687-92.

[8] Vuong, C; Kocianova, S; Yao, Y; Voyich, JM; Yao, Y; Fischer, ER; DeLeo, FR; Otto M. A crucial role for exopolysaccharide modification in bacterial biofilm formation, immune evasion, and virulence. *J Biol Chem.*, 2004, 279(52),54881-6.

[9] O'Riordan, K; Lee, JC. *Staphylococcus aureus* capsular polysaccharides. *Clin Microbiol Rev.*, 2004, 17(1), 218-34.

[10] Gemmell, CG; Tree, R; Patel, A; O'Reilly, M; Foster, TJ. Susceptibility to opsonophagocytosis of protein A, alpha-haemolysin and beta-toxin deficient mutants of *Staphylococcus aureus* isolated by allele-replacement. *Zentbl Bakteriol.*, 1991, 21 (Suppl.), 273-7.

[11] Schlievert, PM. Role of superantigens in human disease. *J Infect Dis.*, 1993, 167(5), 997-1002.

[12] Schlievert, PM; Case, LC. Molecular analysis of staphylococcal superantigens. *Methods Mol Biol.*, 2007, 391, 113-26.

[13] Bubeck, WJ; Schneewind, O. Vaccine protection against *Staphylococcus aureus* pneumonia. *J Exp Med.*, 2008, 205(2), 287-94.

[14] Kaneko, J; Kamio, Y. Bacterial two-component and hetero-heptameric pore-forming cytolytic toxins: structures, pore-forming mechanism, and organization of the genes. *Biosci Biotechnol Biochem.*, 2004, 68(5), 981-1003.

[15] Boyle-Vavra, S; Daum, RS. Community-acquired methicillin-resistant *Staphylococcus aureus*: the role of Panton-Valentine leukocidin. *Lab Invest.*, 2007, 87(1), 3-9.

[16] Wang, R; Braughton, KR; Kretschmer et al. Identification of novel cytolytic peptides as key virulence determinants for community-associated MRSA. *Nat Med.*, 2007, 13(12), 1510-4.

[17] Stefani, S; Chung, DR; Lindsay, JA; Friedrich, AW; Kearns, AM; Westh, H; MacKenzie, FM. Meticillin-resistant *Staphylococcus aureus* (MRSA): global epidemiology and harmonisation of typing methods. *Intl J of Antimicrob Agents.*, 2012, 39(4), 273-82.

[18] Sievert, DM; Ricks, P; Edwards, JR; Schneider, A; Patel, J; Srinivasan, A; Kallen, A; Limbago, B; Fridkin, S. Antimicrobial-Resistant Pathogens Associated with Healthcare-Associated Infections: Summary of Data Reported to the National Healthcare Safety Network at the Centers for Disease Control and Prevention, 2009–2010. *Infect Control Hosp Epidemiol.*, 2013, 34 (1), 1-14.

[19] Pereira, VC; Martins, A; Rugolo, LMSS; Cunha, MLRS. Detection of oxacillin resistance in *Staphylococcus aureus* isolated from the neonatal and pediatric units of a brazilian teaching hospital. *Clin Med Pediatr.*, 2009, 3, 23-31, 2009.

[20] Martins, A; Pereira, VC; Cunha, MLRS. Oxacillin resistance of *Staphylococcus aureus* isolated from the Universtity Hospital of Botucatu Medical School in Brazil. *Chemoterapy.*, 2010, 56(2), 112-9.

[21] Chen, X; Yang, H; Huangfu, Y; Wang, W; Liu, Y; Ni, Y; Han, L. Molecular epidemiologic analysis of *Staphylococcus aureus* isolated from four burn centers. *Burns.*, 2012, 38(5), 738-42.

[22] Machado, ABMP; Reiter, K; Paiva, RM; Barth, AL. Distribution of staphylococcal cassette chromosome *mec* (SCC*mec*) types I, II, III and IV in coagulase-negative staphylococci from patients attending a tertiary hospital in southern *Brazil. J Med Microbiol.*, 2007, 56(Pt10), 1328-33.

[23] Turnidge, J; Grayson, ML. Optimum treatment of staphylococcal infections. *Drugs.*, 1993, 45(3), 353-66.

[24] Chambers, HF. Methicillin resistance in *staphylococci*: molecular and biochemical basis and clinical implications. *Clin Microbiol Rev.*, 1997, 10(4), 781-91.

[25] Hiramatsu, K; Hanaki, H; Ino, T; Yabuta, K; Oguri, T; Tenover, FC. Methicillin-resistant *Staphylococcus aureus* clinical strain with reduced vancomycin susceptibility. *J Antimicrob Chemother.*,1997, 40(1), 135-6.

[26] Wertheim, HF; Melles, DC; Vos, MC; van Leeuwen, W; van Belkum, A; Verbrugh, HA; et al. The role of nasal carriage in *Staphylococcus aureus* infections. *Lancet Infect Dis.*, 2005, 5(12), 751-62.

[27] van Belkum, A; van Leeuwen, W; Kaufmann, ME; Cookson, B; Forey, F; Etienne, J; et al. Assessment of resolution and intercenter reproducibility of results of genotyping *Staphylococcus aureus* by pulsed-field gel electrophoresis of SmaI macrorestriction fragments: a multicenter study. *J Clin Microbiol.*, 1998, 36(6),1653-9.

[28] Frénay, HM; Bunschoten, AE; Schouls, LM; van Leeuwen, WJ; Vandenbroucke-Grauls, CM; Verhoef, J; et al. Molecular typing of methicillin-resistant *Staphylococcus aureus* on the basis of protein A gene polymorphism. *Eur J Clin Microbiol Infect Dis.*, 1996, 15(1), 60-4.

[29] Harmsen, D; Claus, H; Witte, W; Rothgänger, J; Turnwald, D; Vogel, U. Typing of methicillin-resistant *Staphylococcus aureus* in a university hospital setting by using novel software for spa repeat determination and database management. *J Clin Microbiol.*, 2003, 41 (12), 5442-8.

[30] Friedrich, AW; Witte, W; Harmsen, D; de Lencastre, H; Hryniewicz, W; Scheres, J; et al. SeqNet.org: a European laboratory network for sequence-based typing of microbial pathogens. *Euro Surveill.*, 2006, 11(1), E060112.4.

[31] Aires de Sousa, M; de Lencastre, H. Bridges from hospitals to the laboratory: genetic portraits of methicillin-resistant *Staphylococcus aureus* clones. *FEMS Immunol Med Microbiol.*, 2004, 40(2), 101-11.

[32] Church, D; Elsayed, S; Reid, O; Winston, B; Lindsay, R. Burn wound infections. *Clin Microbiol Rev.*, 2006, 19,403-34.

[33] Greenhalgh, DG; Saffle, JR; Holmes, JH; Gamelli, RL; Palmieri, TL; Horton, JW; Tompkins, RG; Traber, DL; Mozingo, DW; Deitch, EA; Goodwin, CW; Herndon, DN; Gallagher, JJ; Sanford, AP; Jeng, JC; Ahrenholz, DH; Neely, AN; O'Mara, MS; Wolf, SE; Purdue, GF; Garner, WL; Yowler, CJ; Latenser, BA. American Burn Association Consensus Conference on Burn Sepsis and Infection Group. American Burn Association consensus conference to define sepsis and infection in burns. *J BurnCare Res.*, 2007, 28, 776-90.

[34] Murray, CK. Burns. In: Bennet JE, Dolin R, Blaser MJ. Mandell, D and Bennett's, editors. *Principles and Practice of Infections Diseases*. 8th. Ed. Philadelphia (PA): Elsevier Saunders, 2015.

[35] Rex, S. Burn injuries. *Curr Opin Crit Care.*, 2012, 18, 671-6.

[36] Rowan, MP; Cancio, LC; Elster, EA; Burmeister, DM; Rose, LF; Natesan, S; Chan, RK; Christy, RJ; Chung, KK. Burn wound healing and treatment: review and advancements. *Crit Care.*, 2015, 19, 243.

[37] Uppal, SK; Ram, S; Kwatra, B; Garg, S; Gupta, R. Comparative evaluation of surface swab and quantitative full thickness wound biopsyculture in burn patients. *Burns*, 2007, 33, 460-3.
[38] Kallstrom, G. Are Quantitative Bacterial Wound Cultures Useful? *J Clin Microbiol.*, 2014, 52, 2753-6.
[39] Steer, JA; Papini, RPR; P, Papini; Wilson, AP; McGrouther, DA; Parkhouse, N. Quantitative microbiology in the management of burn patients. I. Correlation between quantitative and qualitative burn wound biopsy culture and surface alginate swab culture. *Burns*, 1996, 22,173-176.
[40] Rafla, K; Tredget, EE. Infection control in the burn unit. *Burns*. 2011, 37, 5-15.
[41] Toscano Olivo, TE; de Melo, EC; Rocha, C; Fortaleza, CM. Risk factors for acquisition of Methicillin-resistant *Staphylococcus aureus* among patients from a burn unit in Brazil. *Burns*. 2009, 35, 1104-11.
[42] Rodrigues, MV; Fortaleza, CM; Riboli, DF; Rocha, RS; Rocha, C; Cunha, MLRS. Molecular epidemiology of methicillin-resistant *Staphylococcus aureus* in a burn unit from Brazil. *Burns*. 2013, 39, 1242-9.
[43] Avni, T; Levcovich, A; Ad-El, DD; Leibovici, L; Paul, M. Prophylactic antibiotics for burns patients: systematic review and meta-analysis. *BMJ.*, 2010, 340,c241.
[44] Norbury, W; Herndon, DN; Tanksley, J; Jeschke, MG; Finnerty, CC. Infection in Burns. *Surg Infect* (Larchmt). 2016, 17, 250-5.
[45] Posluszny, JA Jr; Conrad, P; Halerz, M; Shankar, R; Gamelli, RL. Surgical burn wound infections and their clinical implications. *J BurnCare Res.*, 2011, 32, 324-33.
[46] Dudeck, MA; Horan, TC; Peterson, KD; Bridson, KA; Morrell, GC; Pollock, DA; Edwards, JR. National Healthcare Safety Network (NHSN) Report, Data Summary for 2009, Device-associated Module. *Am J Infect Control.*, 2011, 39, 349-67.
[47] Rogers, AD; Argent, A;, Rode, H. Review article: ventilator-associated pneumonia in major burns. *Ann Burns Fire Disasters.*, 2012, 25, 135-9.
[48] Lachiewicz, AM; van Duin, D; DiBiase, LM; Jones, SW; Carson, S; Rutala, WA; Cairns, BA; Weber, DJ. Rates of hospital-associated respiratory infections and associated pathogens in a regional burn center, 2008-2012. *Infect Control Hosp Epidemiol*. 2015, 36, 601-3.

[49] Öncül, O; Öksüz, S; Acar, A; Ülkür, E; Turhan, V; Uygur, F; Ulçay, A; Erdem, H; Özyurt, M; Görenek, L. Nosocomial infection characteristics in a burn intensive care unit: analysis of an eleven-year active surveillance. *Burns.* 2014, 40, 835-41.

[50] Al Ashry, HS; Mansour, G; Kalil, AC; Walters, RW; Vivekanandan, R. Incidence of ventilator associated pneumonia in burn patients with inhalation injury treated with high frequency percussive ventilation versus volume control ventilation: A systematic review. *Burns.* 2016 Mar 26. pii: S0305-4179(16)00084-X. doi: 10.1016/j.burns.2016. 02.024. [Epubaheadofprint]

[51] Klompas, M; Kleinman, K; Murphy, MV. Descriptive epidemiology and attributable morbidity of ventilator associated events. *Infect Control Hosp Epidemiol.*, 2014, 35, 502-10.

[52] Klompas, M; Anderson, D; Trick, W; Babcock, H; Kerlin, MP; Li, L; Sinkowitz-Cochran, R; Ely, EW; Jernigan, J; Magill, S; Lyles, R; O'Nei,l C; Kitch, BT; Arrington, E; Balas, MC; Kleinman, K; Bruce, C; Lankiewicz, J; Murphy, MV, Cox, C; Lautenbach, E; Sexton, D; Fraser, V; Weinstein, RA; Platt, R; CDC Prevention Epicenters. The preventability of ventilator-associated events. The CDC Prevention Epicenters Wake Up and Breathe Collaborative. *Am J Respir Crit Care Med.*, 2015, 191, 292-301.

[53] Ottosen, J; Evans, H. Pneumonia: challenges in the definition, diagnosis, and management of disease. *Surg Clin North Am.*, 2014, 94, 1305-17.

[54] Remington, L; Faraklas, I; Gauthier, K; Carper, C; Wiggins, JB; Lewis, GM; Cochran A. Assessment of a Central Line-Associated Bloodstream Infection Prevention Program in a Burn-Trauma Intensive Care Unit. *JAMA Surg.*, 2015, 23, 1-2.

[55] Evans, O; Gowardman, J; Rabbolini, D; McGrail, M; Rickard, CM. In situ diagnostic methods for catheter related blood stream infection in burns patients: A pilot study. *Burns.*, 2016, 42, 434-40.

[56] Raad, I; Hanna, H; Maki, D. Intravascular catheter-related infections: advances in diagnosis, prevention, and management. *Lancet Infect Dis.*, 2007, 7, 645-57.

[57] Christ-Libertin, C; Black, S; Latacki, T; Bair, T. Evidence-based prevent catheter-associated urinary tract infections guidelines and burn-injured patients: a pilot study. *J Burn Care Res.*, 2015, 36, e1-6.

[58] Rodvold, KA; McConeghy, KW. Methicillin-resistant *Staphylococcus aureus* therapy: past, present, and future. *Clin Infect Dis.,* 201, 58, Suppl 1, S20-7.
[59] Rubinstein, E; Keynan, Y. Vancomycin revisited - 60 years later. *Front Public Health.* 2014, 2, 217.
[60] Gardete, S; Tomasz, A. Mechanisms of vancomycin resistance in *Staphylococcus aureus*. *J Clin Invest.,* 2014,124, 2836-40.
[61] Park, SY; Oh, IH; Lee, HJ; Ihm, CG; Son, JS; Lee, MS; Kim MN. Impact of reduced vancomycin MIC on clinical outcomes of methicillin-resistant *Staphylococcus aureus* bacteremia. *Antimicrob Agents Chemother.,* 2013, 57,5536-42.
[62] Casapao, AM; Davis, S; McRoberts, JP; Lagnf, AM; Patel, S; Kullar, R; Levine, DP; Rybak, MJ. Evaluation of vancomycin population susceptibility analysis profile as a predictor of outcomes for patients with infective endocarditis due to methicillin-resistant *Staphylococcus aureus*. *Antimicrob Agents Chemother.,* 2014,58,4636-41.
[63] Chen, CP; Liu, MF; Lin, CF; Lin, SP; Shi, ZY. The association of molecular typing, vancomycin MIC, and clinical outcome for patients with methicillin-resistant *Staphylococcus aureus* infections. *J Microbiol Immunol Infect.,* 2015,pii: S1684-1182(15)00838-5. doi: 10.1016/ j.jmii.2015.08.015. [Epubaheadofprint].
[64] Álvarez, R; López Cortés, LE; Molina, J; Cisneros, JM; Pachón, J. Vancomycin: optimizing its clinical use. *Antimicrob Agents Chemother.,* 2016, pii: AAC.03147-14. [Epubaheadofprint].
[65] Yue, J; Dong, BR; Yang, M; Chen, X; Wu, T; Liu, GJ. Linezolid versus vancomycin for skin and soft tissue infections. *Cochrane Database Syst Rev.,* 2016, 1CD008056.
[66] Wunderink, RG; Niederman, MS; Kollef, MH; Shorr, AF; Kunkel, MJ; Baruch, A; McGee, WT; Reisman, A; Chastre, J. Linezolid in methicillin-resistant *Staphylococcus aureus* nosocomial pneumonia: a randomized, controlled study. *Clin Infect Dis.,* 2012, 54, 621-9.
[67] Kalil, AC; Klompas, M; Haynatzki, G; Rupp, ME. Treatment of hospital-acquired pneumonia with linezolid or vancomycin: a systematic review and meta-analysis. B*MJ Open.,* 2013,3e003912.
[68] Wang, Y; Zou, Y; Xie, J; Wang, T; Zheng, X; He, H; Dong, W; Xing, J; Dong, Y. Linezolid versus vancomycin for the treatment of suspected methicillin-resistant *Staphylococcus aureus* nosocomial pneumonia: a systematic review employing meta-analysis. *Eur J ClinPharmacol.,* 201,71,107-15.

[69] Vilhena, C; Bettencourt, A. Daptomycin: a review of properties, clinical use, drug delivery and resistance. *Mini Rev Med Chem.*, 2012, 12,202-9.
[70] Frampton, JE. Ceftaroline fosamil: a review of its use in thetreatment of complicated skinand soft tissue infections and community-acquired pneumonia. *Drugs.*, 2013, 73(10), 1067-94.
[71] Liapikou, A; Cillóniz, C; Torres, A. Ceftobiprole for the treatment of pneumonia: a European perspective. *Drug Des Devel Ther.*, 2015, 9, 4565-72.
[72] Holmes, NE; Tong, SY; Davis, JS; van Hal, SJ. Treatment of methicillin-resistant *Staphylococcus aureus*: vancomycin and beyond. *Semin Respir Crit Care Med.*, 2015, 36, 17-30.
[73] Van Eperen, AS; Segreti, J. Empirical therapy in Methicillin-resistant *Staphylococcus aureus* infections: An Up-To-Date approach. *J Infect Chemother.*, 2016, pii: S1341-321X(16)30009-5. doi: 10.1016/j.jiac.2016.02.012. [Epubaheadofprint].
[74] HIPAC/IDSA (Healthcare Infection Control Practices Advisory Committee and Hand-HygieneTask Force; Society for Healthcare Epidemiology of America; Association for Professionals in Infection Control and Epidemiology; Infection Diseases Society of America). Guideline for hand hygiene in healthcare settings. *J Am Coll Surg.*, 2004, 198, 121-7.
[75] WHO (World Health Organization). *WHO Guidelines on Hand Hygiene in Health Care: First Global Patient Safety Challenge Clean Care Is Safer Care.* WHO: Geneva, 2009.
[76] Humphreys, H. Do guidelines for the prevention and control of methicillin-resistant *Staphylococcus aureus* make a difference? *Clin Microbiol Infect.*, 2009, 15 Suppl 7, 39-43.
[77] Siegel, JD; Rhinehart, E; Jackson, M; Chiarello, L; Health Care Infection Control Practices Advisory Committee. *Guideline for Isolation Precautions: Preventing Transmission of Infectious Agents in Health Care Settings.* Am J Infect Control., 2007,35 Suppl 2, S65-164.
[78] Clock, SA; Cohen, B; Behta, M; Ross, B; Larson, EL. Contact precautions for multidrug-resistant organisms: Current recommendations and actual practice. *Am J Infect Control.*, 2010, 38, 105-11.
[79] Dokter, J; Brusselaers, N; Hendriks, WD; Boxma, H. Bacteriological cultures on admission of the burn patient: To do or not to do, that's the question. *Burns.*, 2016, 42(2), 421-7.

[80] Johnson, AT; Nygaard, RM; Cohen, EM; Fey, RM; Wagner, AL. The Impact of Hospital-Acquired Methicillin-Resistant *Staphylococcus aureus* in a Burn Population After Implementation of Universal Decolonization Protocol. *J Burn Care Res*., 2015,. [Epubaheadofprint].

[81] Aboelatta, YA; Abd-Elsalam, AM; Omar, AH; Abdelaal, MM; Farid, AM. Selective digestive decontamination (SDD) as a tool in the management of bacterial translocation following major burns. *Ann Burns Fire Disasters*., 2013,26,182-8.

In: *Staphylococcus aureus*
Editor: M. L. R. S. Cunha

ISBN: 978-1-63485-959-2
© 2017 Nova Science Publishers, Inc.

*Chapter 2*

# COMMUNITY-ASSOCIATED *STAPHYLOCOCCUS AUREUS* (CA-MRSA) IN SPECIAL GROUPS

*Camila Sena Martins de Souza,*
*Nathalia Bibiana Teixeira and*
*Maria de Lourdes Ribeiro de Souza da Cunha*[*]
Department of Microbiology and Immunology, Botucatu Institute of
Biosciences, UNESP - Univ Estadual Paulista, Botucatu,
São Paulo State, Brazil

## ABSTRACT

*Staphylococcus aureus* is one of the pathogens most isolated in infections both in hospitals and in the community and it is a major problem for public health systems as it easily acquires resistance to the antimicrobials used. These bacteria are responsible for a wide variety of infections affecting the superficial tissues and also the deepest ones which are penetrated through the disruption of natural barriers. Due to this characteristic, they are associated to skin and soft tissue diseases, serious infections such as toxic shock syndrome, and sepsis, which are all conditions that can be fatal. In 1961, there were the first records of methicillin-resistant *S. aureus* (MRSA) and until the 1990s it was thought

---

[*] Corresponding author: cunhamlr@ibb.unesp.br

to be a nosocomial pathogen called HA-MRSA (*Health-Care-associated Methicillin-Resistant Staphylococcus aureus*) which caused serious infections in individuals with risk factors related to health care. However, its transmission in the community among individuals without risk factors has been reported in the last years, and in this context isolates with specific genetic characteristics, called CA-MRSA (*Community-associated Methicillin-Resistant Staphylococcus aureus*), have been identified. The transmission has occurred easily among detainees, athletes, military soldiers, men who have sex with men, injecting drug users, people with compromised mucous and skin, those with poor hygiene habits, and also children in nurseries due to their contact with contaminated nasal secretions. Some common factors of this spread are crowds, physical skin-to-skin contact with infectious lesions or skin damage, indiscriminate use of antibiotics, sharing personal items that may be contaminated and coming in contact with damaged skin, and also poor practice of hygiene rules, such as lack of hand washing that can lead to the transmission of the bacteria in places like prisons. More recently, long-term care facilities (LTCFs) have been recognized as reservoirs of this pathogen more and more often, probably due to the old patients' age, their lifestyle, need for invasive devices, the presence of chronic wounds, and their dependence on health workers and previous hospitalization. All of these result in many cases of MRSA colonization which remain unrecognized and lead to a spread among the elderly, family members, and health professionals because of their direct contact with them. In addition, the elderly are hospitalized more often and they can be a source of such microorganisms both in hospitals and in the community. People who have HIV/AIDS (PVHA) also have a higher risk of *S. aureus* colonization and therefore of infections such as bacteremia, endocarditis and skin infections. *S. aureus* has also been responsible for the colonization of insulin-dependent diabetics, which increases the predisposition of such individuals to the development of serious infections. Keeping *S. aureus* under control in hospitals and in the community is a major public health concern that is highlighted by the continuing evolution of MRSA. This chapter will address the CA-MRSA in special groups such as PVHA, detainees, the elderly and diabetic patients showing the genetic profile, virulence characteristics and resistance pattern of these isolates aiming at better understanding its epidemiological profile and its impact on the community.

# INTRODUCTION

*Staphylococcus aureus* (*S. aureus*) it stands out as the etiologic agent for presenting relevant morbidity and mortality rates both in hospitals and in the community [1]. It receives attention for its pathogenicity and high frequency, causing disease in both immunocompromised and healthy individuals through its easy intra-hospital dissemination and enormous adaptability and resistance to antibiotics [2].

Nasal colonization by *S. aureus*, as previously mentioned, is devoid of symptoms, i.e., the individual does not develop infection. This asymptomatic colonization has great clinical importance, since, with colonized nostrils, the individual contaminates their own hands and becomes a vehicle for transfer of bacteria via the mechanism of infection through contact [3].

*S. aureus* is one of the most isolated pathogens, both in hospital infections and the community, with high morbidity and mortality, representing a major problem for public health systems [4]. *S. aureus* infections reach from superficial to deeper tissues where they penetrate through the natural barriers and can be associated with skin and soft tissue disease, or serious infections such as endocarditis, pneumonia, meningitis, toxic shock syndrome and sepsis, which can lead to death [1, 5, 6].

In 1961 the first reports of *S. aureus* resistant to methicillin (MRSA) appeared, which until the 1990s was considered a nosocomial pathogen known as HA-MRSA *(Health-Care-associated Methicillin-Resistant Staphylococcus aureus)*, with a limited number of clones causing serious infections in individuals with risk factors associated with health care. However, the transmission in the community between individuals without risk factors has been reported in recent years. In this context, the identification was isolated with specific genetic characteristics, denominated CA-MRSA *(Community-associated Methicillin-Resistant Staphylococcus aureus)* [7].

Epidemiologically, CA-MRSA strains can be defined as clinical isolates of MRSA, collected from ambulatory patients without a history of recent hospitalization or surgery, who have not used intravenous and cutaneous long-term medical devices or catheters in the previous year, or clinical isolates collected from hospital patients within 48h after admission [8, 9].

The emergence of MRSA strains is an important challenge in staphylococcal therapy since these strains are predominantly resistant to all beta-lactams. Beta-lactam antibiotics target the penicillin binding proteins (PBPs), membrane proteins involved in the biosynthesis of the bacterial cell wall. The beta-lactams which interact with PBPs prevent the complete formation of the peptidoglycan layer, triggering bacterial death. However, in the presence of the *mecA* gene, alterations occur in the binding proteins through the encoding of a new target protein, termed PBP 2a, which presents a low affinity for beta-lactams. The beta-lactam antibiotics used clinically do not bind to PBP 2a in therapeutic concentrations and therefore lead to a lack of efficacy against infections caused by MRSA [10, 11].

The *mecA* gene is located in a movable genetic complex called *Staphylococcal Cassette Chromosome mec* (SCC*mec*). To date, eleven types of SCC*mec* have been described for *S. aureus,* using the combination of two parts: the *ccr* complex and the *mec* complex, with three phylogenetically distinct *ccr* genes, classified as *ccrA*, *ccrB* and *ccrC*. Furthermore, there are six classes in the *mec* gene complex (class A, B, C1, C2, D and E); at the moment in class D there are no described SCC*mec* [11, 12].

The different types of SCC*mec* are classified as: SCC*mec* type I (*mec* complex gene class *B* and *ccrA1B1*), SCC*mec* type II (*mec* complex gene class *A* and *ccrA2B2*), SCC*mec* type III (*mec* complex gene class *A* and *ccrA3B3*), SCC*mec* type IV (*mec* complex gene class *B* and *ccrA2B2*), SCC*mec* type V (*mec* complex gene class *C2* and *ccrC*), SCC*mec* type VI (*mec* complex gene class *B* and *ccrA4B4*), SCC*mec* type VII (*mec* complex gene class *C1* and *ccrC*), SCC*mec* type VIII (*mec* complex gene class *A* and *ccrA4B4*), SCC*mec* type IX (*mec* complex gene class *C2* and *ccrA1B1*), SCC*mec* type X (*mec* complex gene class *C1* and *ccrA1B6*) and SCC*mec* type XII (*mec* complex gene class *E* and *ccrA1B3*). The remaining region of the *SCCmec* is called the J region (*Joining region*), which possesses non-essential components of the cassette that may carry additional antimicrobial resistance determinants [12].

Despite the difficulty in distinguishing between these strains, CA-MRSA are characterized by presenting greater susceptibility to non-beta-lactam agents, carrying principally SCC*mec* type IV and more frequently possessing the gene for Panton-Valentine leukocidin (PVL) [13].

The incidence of CA-MRSA varies geographically and according to sex and age; to date there have been reports of CA-MRSA affecting young people, adults and children. Transmission occurs easily between inmates, athletes, military recruits, men who have sex with men, injecting drug users, people with compromised skin and mucous membranes and those with poor hygiene habits and between children in day care centers, due to contact with contaminated nasal secretions [14, 15].

Some common factors of this propagation are: concentration of people, physical skin to skin contact with infectious wounds or damaged skin, the indiscriminate use of antibiotics, sharing personal items that may be contaminated and which come into contact with broken skin, as well as poor hygiene practices such as lack of hand washing that can facilitate the transmission of bacteria in environments such as prisons [16].

## SPECIAL GROUPS

More recently, long-term care facilities (LTC) have been increasingly recognized as reservoirs of this pathogen, possibly due to the advanced age of the elderly, lifestyle, the need for invasive devices, the presence of chronic wounds, dependence on health workers and previous hospitalization, resulting in many cases of MRSA colonization that remain unrecognized and lead to the spread among the elderly, their families and health professionals, due to direct contact between them. In addition, the elderly are considered a vulnerable group, admitted to hospitals with greater frequency, and can be source of these microorganisms in the hospital/community interface [17, 18].

Studies have shown that *S. aureus* is an important cause of morbidity among hospitalized patients and have identified that people living with HIV/AIDS (PVHA) have an increased risk of nasopharyngeal colonization with pathogenic microorganisms, principally related to *S. aureus*, and consequently the occurrence of infections, including bacteremia, endocarditis and skin infections [19, 20].

Padoveze et al. [21] suggest that the acquisition of nasal MRSA colonization is related to hospitalization in an infectious diseases unit and frequent health service assistance in daily care clinics for HIV/AIDS patients, demonstrating the need for vigilance in clinics, due to the possible implications of the spread of resistant organisms, such as MRSA.

Some studies report that the combination of low levels of CD4+T lymphocytes leads to a greater risk of infection with MRSA and suggest that this may be increased by immunodeficiency. Among the risk factors found for the initial development of MRSA infections in PVHA patients are frequent exposure to antibiotics, sociodemographic, behavioral and psychosocial factors, such as high risk sexual behavior, the use of illicit drugs, hospitalizations, contact with health professionals and weakened immune status, among others, which play an important role in increasing the risk of MRSA infection and the establishment of higher rates of colonization among this patient population [22, 23, 24].

The prevalence of carriers with *S. aureus* can vary according to the population studied. It is recognized that individuals who frequently use needles, either for insulin or drug use present higher rates than other individuals, ranging from 24.1% to 76.4%, with a mean of 56.4% [25]. Studies have demonstrated that the rate of nasal colonization by *S. aureus* is higher in diabetic patients than in non-diabetics [26] and that diabetes is a major risk factor for colonization and infection with MRSA.

Diabetic patients are prone to persistent infections, especially skin infections such as those caused by *S. aureus,* due to increased blood glucose levels and suppression of the immune response. Moreover, the presence of slow healing wounds is very common in these patients, due to the presence of neuropathies and decreased blood flow to the extremities [27]. These infections are generally recognized as frequent causes of morbidity and mortality among diabetic patients. According to health ministry data [28], every ten seconds a person dies in the world as a result of complications of diabetes, 3.2 million deaths per year.

Currently, programs for the control and prevention of infectious diseases observed in several countries have increased their efforts to reduce the transmission of *S. aureus* and MRSA through the implementation of a series of measures to control the infection. Hand hygiene, both for health professionals, who constitute the main vehicle for transmission of MRSA, and individuals in contact with patients, has been a primary containment measure for reducing transmission [29, 30]. The characterization of strains and decolonization of individuals may be useful tools to contain outbreaks caused by CA-MRSA which can be used in high prevalence areas or critical situations, however this is controversial. Existing nasal decolonization protocols for patients and health professionals who are MRSA carriers, adopt the use of mupirocin (topical nasal antibiotic) and skin decolonization with daily chlorhexidine bathing, however this technique is not consensual, since *S. aureus* is known for its high potential to develop resistance, and the risk of re-colonization cannot be ruled out [30].

Controlling and understanding *S. aureus,* in both hospital and community environments, is a major public health concern, highlighted by the continuing evolution and development of MRSA.

It is worth mentioning that the presence of MSSA (Methicillin Susceptible *Staphylococcus aureus*) is also of great relevance for possessing virulence factors that enhance its invasiveness and survival, leading to a greater ability to disseminate, and the fact that these microorganisms are the likely source of MRSA strains through the acquisition of resistance determinants such as the *mecA* gene, present in the mobile genetic element known as SCC*mec*.

## REFERENCES

[1] Edwards, AM; Massey, RC; Clarke, SR. Molecular mechanisms of *Staphylococcus aureus* nasopharyngeal colonization. *Mol Oral Microbiol.*, 2012, 27(1), 1-10.

[2] Otto, M. 2010. Basis of Virulence in Community-Associated Methicillin-Resistant *Staphylococcus aureus*. *Annu Rev Microbiol.*, 2010, 64, 143–62.

[3] Santos, AL; Santos, DO; Freitas, CC; Ferreira, BLA; Afonso, IF; Rodrigues, CR; Castro, HC. 2007. *Staphylococcus aureus*: visitando uma cepa de importância hospitalar. *J Bras Patol Med Lab.*, 2007, 43(6), 413-23.

[4] Chen, FJ; Huang, IW; Wang, CH; Chen, PC; Wang, HY; Lai, JF; Shiau, YR; Lauderdale, TY; TSAR Hospitals. *mecA*-Positive *Staphylococcus aureus* with low-level oxacillin MIC in Taiwan. *J Clin Microbiol.*, 2012, 50(5), 1679-83.

[5] Li, M; DX; Villaruz, AE; Diep, BA; Wang, D; Song, Y; Tian, Y; Hu, J; Yu, F; Lu, Y; Otto, M. MRSA epidemic linked to a quickly spreading colonization and virulence determinant. *Nad Med.*, 2012, 18(5), 816-9.

[6] Adhikari, RP; Ajao, AO; Aman, JM; Karauzum, H; Sarwar J; Lydecker, AD; Johnson, KJ; Nguyen, C; Chen, WH; Roghmann, MC. Lower antibody levels to *Staphylococcus aureus* exotoxins are associated with sepsis in hospitalized adults with invasive *S. aureus* infections. *J Infect Dis.*, 2012, 206(6), 915-23.

[7] Mediavilla, JR; Chen, L; Mathema, B; Kreiswirthet, BN. Global epidemiology of community-associated methicillin resistant *Staphylococcus aureus* (CA-MRSA). *Curr Opin Microbiol.*, 2012, 15(5), 588-95.

[8] Gelatti, LC; Bonamigo, RR; Becker, AP; d´Azevedo, PA. *Staphylococcus aureus* resistentes à meticilina: disseminação emergente na comunidade. *An Bras Dermatol.*, 2009, 84(5), 501-6.

[9] Yamamoto, T; Hung, WC; Takano, T; Nishiyama, A. Genetic nature and virulence of community associated methicillin-resistant *Staphylococcus aureus*. *Biomed.*, 2013, 3(1), 1-17.

[10] Katayama, Y; Zhang, HZ; Chambers, HF. PBP 2a mutations producing very high-level resistance to beta-lactams. *Antimicrob Agents Chemother.*, 2004, 48(2), 453-9.

[11] Monecke, S; Coombs, G; Shore, AC, Coleman, DC; Akpaka, P; Borg, M; Chow, H; Ip, M; Jatzwauk, L; Jonas, D; Kadlec, K; Kearns, A; Laurent, F; O'Brien, FG; Pearson, J; Ruppelt, A; Schwarz, S; Scicluna, E; Slickers, P; Tan, HL; Weber, S; Ehricht, R. A Field Guide to Pandemic, Epidemic and Sporadic Clones of Methicillin-Resistant *Staphylococcus aureus*. *Plos One*, 2011, 6(4), 1793-6.

[12] (IWG-SCC) International Working Group on the Classification of Staphylococcal Cassete Chromosome Elements. Classification of staphylococcal cassette chromosome *mec* (SCC*mec*): guidelines for reporting novel SCC*mec* elements. *Antimicrob Agents Chemother.* 2009, 53(12): 4961-7.

[13] Cooke, FJ; Brown, NM. Community-associated methicillin-resistant *Staphylococcus aureus* infections. *Brit Med Bul.*, 2010, 94, 215-27.

[14] CDC. *Centers for Disease Control and Prevention. Staphylococcus aureus* resistant to vancomycin-United States. *Morb Mortal. Wkly Rep*, 2002, 51, 565–7.

[15] CDC. *Centers for Disease Control and Prevention*. Methicillin-resistant *Staphylococcus aureus* infections among competitive sports participants-Colorado, Indiana, Pennsylvania, and Los Angeles County, 2000-2003. *Morb Mortal Wkly Rep*, 2003, 52, 793-5.

[16] Cohen, PR. Cutaneous community-acquired methicillin resistant *Staphylococcus aureus* infection in participants of athletic activities. *South Med J.*, 2005, 98(6), 506-602.

[17] Pfingsten-Würzburg S; Pieper DH; Bautsch W; Probst-Kepper M. Prevalence and molecular epidemiology of meticillin- resistant *Staphylococcus aureus* in nursing home residents in northern Germany. *J Hosp Infect.*, 2011, 78(2), 108-12.

[18] Horner C, Parnell P, Hall D, Kearns A, Heritage J, Wilcox M. Methicillin-resistant *Staphylococcus aureus* in elderly residents of care homes: colonization rates and molecular epidemiology. *J Hosp Infect.*, 2013, 83(3), 212-8.

[19] McDonald, C; Lauderdale, TL; Lo, HJ; Tsai, JJ; Hung, CC. Colonization of HIV-infected outpatients in Taiwan with methicillin-resistant and methicillin-susceptible *Staphylococcus aureus*. *Int J STD AIDS.*, 2003, 14(7), 473-7.

[20] Imaz, A; Pujol, M; Barragán, P; Domínguez, MA; Tiraboschi, JM; Podzamczer, D. Community associated methicillin-resistant *Staphylococcus aureus* in HIV-infected patients. *AIDS Reviews.*, 2010, 12(3), 153-63.

[21] Padoveze, MC; Tresoldi, AT; Nowakonski, AV; Aoki, FH; Branchini, MLM. Nasal MRSA Colonization of AIDS Patients Cared for in a Brazilian University Hospital. *Infect Control Hosp Epidemiol.*, 2001, 22(12), 783-5.
[22] Crum-Cianflone, N; Weekes, J; Bavaro, M. Recurrent Community-Associated Methicillin-Resistant *Staphylococcus aureus* Infections among HIV-Infected Persons: Incidence and Risk Factors. AIDS *Patient Care* STDS., 2009, 23(7), 499-502.
[23] Siberry, GK; Frederick, T; Emmanuel, P; Paul, ME; Bohannon, B; Wheeling, T; Barton, T; Rathore, MH; Dominguez, KL. Methicillin-Resistant *Staphylococcus aureus* infections in human immunodeficiency virus-infected children and adolescents. *AIDS Res Treat.*, 2012, 1-7.
[24] Hidron, AL; Kempker, R; Moanna, A; Rimland, D. Methicillin-resistant *Staphylococcus aureus* in HIV-infected patients. *Infect Drug Resist.* 2010, 3, 73–86.
[25] Kluytmans, J; Belkum, AV; Verbrugh, H. Nasal carriage of *Staphylococcus aureus*: epidemiology, underlying mechanisms, and associated risks. *Clin Microbiol Rev.*, 1997, 10(3), 505–20.
[26] Wertheim, HFL; Melles, DC; Vos Margreet, C; van Leeuwen, W; van Belkum, A; Verbrugh, HA; Nouwen, JL. The role of nasal carriage in *Staphylococcus aureus* infections. *The Lancet Infect Dis.*, 2005, 5(12), 751–62.
[27] Trivedi, U; Parameswaran, S; Armstrong, A; Burgueno-Veja, D; Griswold, J; Dissanaike, S; Rumbaugh, KP. Prevalence of Multiple Antibiotic Resistant Infections in Diabetic versus Nondiabetic Wounds. *J Pathog.*, 2014, 1-6.
[28] Ministério da Saúde. 2014. Acessed may 01. http://www.saude.gov.br.
[29] Sousa, MA. *Staphylococcus aureus* resistente à meticilina (MRSA): um pesadelo para a saúde pública. Rev Ciên Saúde., 2012, 4, 18-30.
[30] Sai N; Laurent C; Strale H; Denis O; Byl B. Efficacy of the decolonization of methicillin resistant *Staphylococcus aureus* carriers in clinical practice. *Antimicrob Resist Infect Control.*, 2015, 4(56), 1-8.

In: *Staphylococcus aureus*
Editor: M. L. R. S. Cunha

ISBN: 978-1-63485-959-2
© 2017 Nova Science Publishers, Inc.

*Chapter 3*

# MOLECULAR EPIDEMIOLOGY OF LIVESTOCK-ASSOCIATED METHICILLIN-RESISTANT *STAPHYLOCOCCUS AUREUS* (LA-MRSA)

*Priscila Luiza Mello[1], Luiza Pinheiro[1], Lisiane de Almeida Martins[2] and Maria de Lourdes Ribeiro de Souza da Cunha[1],\**

[1]Department of Microbiology and Immunology, Botucatu Biosciences Institute, UNESP - Univ Estadual Paulista, Botucatu, São Paulo State, Brazil
[2]Universidade Paranaense – UNIPAR, Umuarama – PR, Brazil

## ABSTRACT

Recognized as one of the main causes of human infections worldwide, *Staphylococcus aureus* is also considered a harmful pathogen for veterinary medicine. This microorganism produces a significant number of virulence factors and may acquire resistance to methicillin, giving rise to the so-called methicillin-resistant *S. aureus* (MRSA), which have been considered a health issue for decades. When colonizing hospitalized individuals, MRSA is the main microbial agent related to

---

\* Corresponding author: cunhamlr@ibb.unesp.br

Hospital-Acquired infections (HA-MRSA), being associated to high rates of morbidity, mortality and medical expenses. The epidemiology of MRSA has changed since the emergence of the Community-Acquired MRSA (CA-MRSA), strains that cause infections in healthy individuals. In 2003, a third epidemiological form, the Livestock-Associated MRSA (LA-MRSA), was described first in Netherlands, followed by other countries. The majority of the LA-MRSA isolates have shown to belong to the clonal complex CC398, despite other clonal complexes and *spa* types have been observed. Although related to animal infections, the LA-MRSA strains demonstrate potential to colonize and infect humans, being considered a threat in occupational health, especially for farmers and veterinarians. The zoonotic reservoir for such isolates is believed to be farm animals, mainly swine. The indiscriminate use of antimicrobials in livestock is considered a risk factor for the presence of MRSA; however, the level of hygiene and contact/trading of animals are also important for its dissemination. In 2005, the transmission of LA-MRSA to farmers and their family members in Europe raised the concerns regarding their introduction in the community and hospitals. From 2012 to 2014, four people with no relation to swine production died due to sepsis caused by MRSA CC398 in Denmark, a country that produces around 30 million of swine and is one of the largest exporters in the world. In the Netherlands, the presence of LA-MRSA has been widely investigated in healthy swine, calves, horses and birds, and being described in dairy cattle as cause of subclinical mastitis. Although the infections caused by LA-MRSA in humans may seem unusual, such reservoir may significantly contribute to the raised global dissemination of MRSA. This phenomenon is especially worrying in countries presenting low prevalence of MRSA, since these strains have unexpectedly emerged in Europe and North America. The objective of this chapter is to provide data for a better understanding of the epidemiology and microbial properties of LA-MRSA.

## INTRODUCTION

*Staphylococcus aureus* is one of the most common causes of infections in the world, not only in human but also in veterinary medicine. This microorganism produces a wide range of virulence factors and can also acquire resistance to methicillin, giving rise to methicillin-resistant *Staphylococcus aureus* (MRSA), which have posed a considerable health threat for decades [1].

MRSA can colonize and infect hospitalized individuals or not and are the main pathogens involved in hospital-acquired infections (HA-MRSA), which are characterized by high mortality and increased health expenditure. The epidemiology of MRSA has changed with the emergence of community-associated MRSA (CA-MRSA), which affect healthy individuals without any connection to healthcare facilities [2]. In 2003, a third epidemiological form was recognized, which was called livestock-associated MRSA (LA-MRSA). These microorganisms were identified in The Netherlands and have since then emerged in many other countries [3].

Although LA-MRSA rarely cause infections in animals, they have shown a potential to colonize and infect humans and represent an occupational health risk in which individuals who are in contact with colonized animals are more likely to become colonized/infected [4]. Disease attributed to LA-MRSA in humans seems to be uncommon. However, this reservoir may contribute significantly to the global transport of these microorganisms that emerged throughout Europe and North America in the last decade, especially to countries where the prevalence of LA-MRSA is low. In this respect, food-producing animals are increasingly recognized as an important reservoir of MRSA.

LA-MRSA will be discussed in this chapter in order to provide a better understanding of their microbial properties and epidemiological characteristics.

## CA-MRSA AND HA-MRSA

At present, *Staphylococcus aureus*, particularly MRSA, is one of the most common causes of bacterial infections and the leading pathogen of nosocomial infections [5]. The rates of antimicrobial resistance are increasing, especially those related to hospital deaths. Hospital-associated MRSA (HA-MRSA) strains occur in hospitals and mainly affect immunocompromised patients. These microorganisms have spread globally in hospitals and healthcare facilities since the 1960s and emerged as endemic pathogens in different countries, including the most underdeveloped nations [6].

Deaths caused by MRSA started to increase even among those people who had no connection to hospitals. By 2000, in many countries, most MRSA began to be acquired in the community among people who had no contact with any healthcare facility [7, 8]. These infections are distinguished epidemiologically by the fact that they occur on a large scale in the community and are reported to be caused by community-associated MRSA (CA-MRSA). CA-MRSA strains are a matter of concern since they affect individuals who have no classical risk factors for the development of infection.

## LA-MRSA

The main clonal lineage of LA-MRSA belongs to the clonal complex (CC) 398 and emerged in 2003. The main spa type is T034. Isolate ST398, the first representative of LA-MRSA [9], seems to have emerged independently in the pig population, different from HA-MRSA and CA-MRSA [10]. The LA-MRSA isolates belong to unique lineages that do not spread easily in hospitals [11].

A specific MRSA clone, known as CC398, was detected in pigs in the Netherlands [12] and was subsequently identified in many animal species around the world. Nevertheless, most studies have investigated its prevalence in pigs [12].

Although CC398 is the most prevalent clone among pigs in Europe, other clonal complexes and *spa* types have been observed [13, 14]. Furthermore, methicillin-susceptible *S. aureus* (MSSA) strains that belong to clonal complex CC30 and spa type T1333 have been isolated from pigs [4].

In contrast, in Asia, MRSA CC9 appears as the prevalent clone associated with pig farming [12]. MRSA strains derived from the human lineages ST5, ST8, ST22, ST30 and ST45 have also been described in pigs from Europe, the United States, and Africa [12].

A survey conducted in Belgium comprising the period from 2007 to 2013 determined the prevalence of MRSA in poultry, cattle, and pigs [15]. The study was carried out on different randomly selected pig farms to monitor the epidemiology of LA-MRSA among asymptomatic pigs. The estimated prevalence of MRSA was 65.6%. Similar results have been reported in other studies [16].

## Risk Factors

Although LA-MRSA rarely cause infections in animals, they have shown a potential to colonize and infect humans and represent an occupational health risk. In this respect, individuals who are in contact with colonized animals, such as farmers and veterinarians, are more likely to become colonized/infected. So far, LA-MRSA are prevalent among workers of this risk group [5].

Studies have shown an association between recent contact with food-producing animals and clinical disease resulting from infection with MRSA

CC398 [17, 18]. Thus, as reported for other MRSA strains, LA-MRSA may be responsible for infections in individuals who underwent surgery or hospitalized individuals [19].

The use of antimicrobial agents in animal production is a risk factor for the presence of MRSA. However, other factors such as hygiene and retail/contact with animals are important for their propagation [5]. Food chains are an important route of transmission of microorganisms between animals, including wild animals and humans. The inspection and monitoring of MRSA are therefore recommended worldwide [20].

Studies that detected LA-MRSA in bulk tank milk samples suggested healthy animals or those with subclinical mastitis to play an important role in the dissemination of these strains between animals, workers and the farm environment. Raw milk and milk products are included in the categories of foods that require MRSA monitoring in Europe [21].

Hadjirin et al. [19] published the first report of LA-MRSA CC398 in retail meat products in the United Kingdom. The presence of a lineage that is able to colonize a wide range of host species with a zoonotic potential makes this finding important for both human and animal health. Moreover, the presence of LA-MRSA CC398 in human food products demonstrates, in addition to the established risk through direct contact with food-producing animals, a possible additional pathway for the transmission of antimicrobial resistance from livestock to the general human population and not only to those who have direct contact with farm animals [19]. Adequate cooking (heating above 71°C) of animal foods and hygiene precautions during preparation are recommended to minimize the likelihood of colonization [19].

The occurrence of MRSA in retail meat has been investigated in several European studies and the highest prevalence was found in poultry meat, with CC398 being identified as the most common type [22, 23, 24]. In contrast, a study conducted in the United States reported divergent results. In that study, 289 meat samples (beef, chicken, and turkey) were investigated and MRSA strains were detected in 1.3 to 3.9% of the samples. All isolates belonged to USA300, a finding suggesting human contamination [25].

Although MRSA are found in meats across the world, so far there are no studies showing that meat is a source of human infection. Hence, no evidence exists indicating an increased risk of human colonization or infection after contact or consumption of foods contaminated with CC398 in the community or in hospitals [3].

## EPIDEMIOLOGY

Infection with LA-MRSA is the direct result of the indiscriminate use of antibiotics in livestock farming, including growth promoters [9, 26]. These promoters are aimed at maximizing profit by reducing the time necessary for the animals to reach slaughter weight, thus conferring an economic advantage to the production companies [27]. Growth promoters are also used for the prophylactic treatment of diseases associated with the intensive production of feedlot animals.

The constant exposure to low-dose nontherapeutic antibiotics added to feed or water exerts selective pressures on the survival of resistant pathogens or pathogens with reduced susceptibility [28]. Each animal consuming low levels of antibiotics used as growth promoters may select pathogens that carry resistance genes [29]. Additionally, the larger the number of animals in a feedlot environment, the higher the risk of transmission of bacteria and resistance genes [26, 30]. It is believed that LA-MRSA was originally a human-adapted MSSA, which has adapted to intensively raised pigs and acquired resistance genes as a result of routinely administered antibiotic growth promoters and of the selective pressure created by the use of antimicrobials, permitting the multiplication of resistant strains [31].

LA-MRSA has been detected in food-producing animals (pigs, cattle, and chicken) [32, 33], as well as in horses and pets [34]. The strain belonging to CC398 can also inhabit humans, especially in the case of occupational contact with food-producing animals that carry this strain [35].

Loeffler et al. [36] described the first isolation of LA-MRSA ST398 from retail meat of farms in the United Kingdom. Recent reports of CC398 isolates from horses [37], dairy cattle [38], domestic poultry [41], and pigs [40, 41] indicate that this lineage is widely distributed in the United Kingdom. In many countries, LA-MRSA CC398 represents an occupational risk for people in close contact with animals, especially pigs and veal calves. For example, epidemiological studies have demonstrated significantly higher rates of nasal transmission of MRSA CC398 by humans in contact with pigs (farm workers, abattoir workers, veterinarians) [42]. Cuny et al. [43] isolated 272 MRSA from horses and workers of 17 equine hospitals and 39 veterinary practices in Germany. These isolates were submitted to molecular typing and most isolates from horses were attributed to CC398 (82.7%) and CC8 (16.5%).

The impact of livestock as a reservoir of MRSA for humans is still under investigation. Whereas 23 to 38% of individuals who had contact with MRSA-positive pigs or veal cattle were colonized with these bacteria [44, 45, 46], only 4% of relatives who were not directly exposed to these animals were found to be colonized in another study [47]. In areas with a high density of MRSA CC398-positive pigs, this clone may markedly influence the epidemiology of MRSA in healthcare settings. For example, this strain led to a three-fold increase in the incidence of MRSA over a few years in a Dutch hospital located in an area with a high density of pigs [44]. In a German hospital located in an area with intense livestock farming, 22% of patients colonized with MRSA carried this strain at hospital admission [48].

The transmission of MRSA CC398 from animal reservoirs to hospitals can result in the nosocomial dissemination of MRSA to groups of patients that are susceptible to the development of MRSA infections [49]. The nosocomial transmission of MRSA CC398 has been described [50] and this strain has been associated with cases of severe infections such as endocarditis, soft tissue infections, and ventilation-associated pneumonia [51, 52, 53]. The emergence of human infections caused by MRSA CC398 in Europe remains poorly understood. The proportion of MRSA CC398 among all MRSA ranges from 0.3% in Germany [53] to 41% in The Netherlands [54]. Major concerns include the facts that the genes encoding the cytotoxin Panton–Valentine Leukocidin (PVL) and plasmid *cfr*, which confers resistance to oxazolidinones, were identified in MRSA CC398 strains [55, 56].

## CONCLUSION

The final challenge remains the combat of reservoir animals of MRSA. Despite the Europe-wide dissemination of MRSA in pigs, its implications for humans directly or indirectly exposed to livestock farming and for patients attending health services located in farming areas remain uncertain. Although the epidemic transmission of LA-MRSA among people without direct contact with animals is rare and the emergence of human infections caused by LA-MRSA is still much lower than that caused by CA-MRSA, infection control measures in many European countries should consider the potential risk of acquiring MRSA through contact with livestock farming.

## REFERENCES

[1] Blodkamp, S; Kadlec, K; Gutsmann, T; Naim, HY; Von Köckritz-Blickwede, M; Schwarz, S;. In vitro activity of human and animal cathelicidins against livestock-associated methicillin-resistant *Staphylococcus aureus*. *Vet Microbiol.*, 2015, 1, 1-5.

[2] Hetem, DJ; Derde, LP; Empel, Mroczkowska, GJA; Orczykowska-Kotyna, M; Kozińska, A; Hryniewicz, W; Goossens, H; Bonten, MJM;. Molecular Epidemiology of MRSA in 13 ICUs from eight European Countries. *Antimicrob Chemoter.*, 2015, 1, 45-52.

[3] EFSA. Assessment of the Public Health significance of methicillin resistant *Staphylococcus aureus* (MRSA) in animals and foods; Scientific Opinion of the Panel on Biological Hazards. *EFSA J.*, 2009, 993, 1–7.

[4] Agerso, Y; Hasman, H; Cavaco, LM; Pedersen, K; Aarestrup, FM. Study of methicillin resistant *Staphylococcus aureus* (MRSA) in Danish pigs at slaughter and in imported retail meat reveals a novel MRSA type in slaughter pigs. *Vet Microbiol.*, 2012, 25, 246-250.

[5] Stefani, SDR; Chung, JA; Lindsay, AW; Friedrich, AM; Kearns, H; Westh MacKenzie, FM. Methicillin-resistant *Staphylococcus aureus* (MRSA): global epidemiology and harmonisation of typing methods. *International Journal of Antimicrobial Agents.*, 2012. 39,273– 282.

[6] Graves, SF; Kobayashi, SD; DeLeo, FR. Community-associated methicillin-resistant *Staphylococcus aureus* immune evasion and virulence. *J Mol Med.*, 2010, 88(2),109-114.

[7] Feingold, BJ; Silbergeld, EK; Curriero, FC; Van Cleef, B; Heck, M; Kluytmans, J.. Livestock Density as Risk Factor for Livestock-associated Methicillin-Resistant *Staphylococcus aureus*, the Netherlands. *Emerging Infectious Diseases.*, 2012, 18(11),1841-1849.

[8] Matlow, AS; Forgie, L; Pelude, J; Embree, D; Gravel, JM; Langley, NL; et al. Canadian Nosocomial Infection Surveillance Program. National Surveillance of Methicillin-resistant *Staphylococcus aureus* Among Hospitalized Pediatric Patients in Canadian Acute Care Facilities, 1995–2007. *Pediatr Infect Dis J.*, 2012, 31(8), 814-820.

[9] Hasman, H. 2009. *Staphylococcus aureus* Protein A (spa) Typing [online]. *National Food Institute DTU*. [cited 12 October 2015]. Avaiable from: http://www.eurl-ar.eu/data/images/tc_april-2009/7-8-spa%20and%20mlst_henrik.pdf

[10] McCarthy, AJ; Lindsay, JA; Loeffler, A. 2012. Are all methicillin-resistant *Staphylococcus aureus* (MRSA) equal in all hosts? Epidemiological and genetic comparison between animal and human MRSA. *Veterinary Dermatology.*, 23, 267-275.

[11] Bootsma, MC; Wassenberg, MW; Trapman, P; Bonten, MJ. The nosocomial transmission rate of animal-associated ST398 methicillin-resistant *Staphylococcus aureus*. *J R Soc Interface.*, 2011, 8, 578-584.

[12] Crombé, F; Argudín, MA; Vanderhaeghen, W; Hermans, K; Haesebrouck, F; Butaye, P. Transmission dynamics of methicillin-resistant *Staphylococcus aureus* in pigs. *Front. Microbiol.*, 2013, 4, (57).

[13] Franco, A; Hasman, H; Lurescia, M; Lorenzetti, R; Stegger, M; Pantosti, A; et al. Molecular characterization of spa type t127, sequence type 1 methicillin-resistant *Staphylococcus aureus* from pigs. *J. Antimicrob Chemother.*, 2011, 66, 1231–1235.

[14] Pomba, C; Hasman, H; Cavaco, LM; Fonseca, JD; Aarestrup, FM. First description of meticillin-resistant *Staphylococcus aureus* (MRSA) CC30 and CC398 from swine in Portugal. *Int J Antimicrob Agents.*, 2009, 34,193–194.

[15] Nemeghaire, S; Argudín, MA; Haesebrouck, F; Butaye, P. 2014. Epidemiology and molecular characterization of methicillin-resistant *Staphylococcus aureus* nasal carriage isolates from bovines. *BMC Veterinary Research* 10,153.

[16] Peeters, LEJ; Argudína, MA; Azadikhaha, S; Butayeb, P. Antimicrobial resistance and population structure of *Staphylococcus aureus* recovered from pigs farms. *Vet Microbiology.*, 2015, 180,151–156.

[17] Krziwanek, KS; Metz, G; Mittermayer, H. Methicillin- Resistant *Staphylococcus aureus* ST398 from human patients, upper Austria. *Emerging Inf Dis.*, 2009, 15(5), 766-9.

[18] Aspiroz, C; Lozano, C; Vindel, A; Lasarte, JJ; Zarazaga, M; Torres, C. Skin lesion caused by ST398 and ST1 MRSA, Spain. *Emerging Inf Dis.*, 2010, 16 (1),157-159.

[19] Hadjirin, NF; Lay, EM; Paterson, GK; Harrison, EM; Peacock, SJ; Parkhill, J; Zadoks, RN; Holmes, MA. Detection of livestock-associated methicillin-resistant *Staphylococcus aureus* CC398 in retail pork, United Kingdom. *Euro Surveill.*, 2015, 20(24).

[20] Traversa, A; Gariano, GR; Gallina, S; Bianchi, DM; Orusa, R.; Domenis, L; Cavallerio, P; Fossati, L; Serra, P; Decastelli, L. Methicillin resistance in *Staphylococcus aureus* strains isolated from food and wild animal carcasses in Italy. *Food Microbiology.*, 2015, 52, 154-158.

[21] EFSA (European Food Safety Authority). Technical specifications on the harmonized monitoring and reporting of antimicrobial resistance in methicillin resistant *Staphylococcus aureus* in food-producing animals and food. *EFSA J.*, 2012, 10 (10), 2897.

[22] De Boer, E; Zwartkruis-Nahuis, JT; Wit, B; Huijsdens, XW; De Neeling, AJ; Bosch, T; Van Oosterom, RA; Vila, A; Heuvelink, AE. Prevalence of methicillin-resistant *Staphylococcus aureus* in meat. *Int J Food Microbiol.*, 2009, 134, 52-56.

[23] Fessler, AT; Kadlec, K; Hassel, M; Hauschild, T; Eidam, C; Ehricht, R; Monecke, S; Schwarz, S. Characterization of methicillin-resistant *Staphylococcus aureus* isolates from food and food products of poultry origin in Germany. Appl. Environ. *Microbiol.*, 2011, 77, 7151–7157.

[24] Lozano, C; Lopez, M; Gomez-Sanz, E; Ruiz-Larrea, F.; Torres, C; Zarazaga, M. Detection of methicillin-resistant *Staphylococcus aureus* ST398 in food samples of animal origin in Spain. *J Antimicrob Chemother.*, 2009. 64,1325–1326.

[25] Bhargava, K; Wang, X; Donabedian, S; Zervos, M; de Rocha, L; Zhang, Y. Methicillin-resistant *Staphylococcus aureus* in retail meat, Detroit, MI, USA. *Emerg Infect Dis.*, 2011, 17, 1135–1137.

[26] Greenen, PL; Koene, MGJ; Blaak, H; Havelaar, AH; Van de Giessen, AW. Risk profile on antimicrobial resistance transmissible from food animals to humans. *National Institute for Public Health and the Environment.*, 2010, 1-118.

[27] Croft, AC; D'Antoni, AV; Terzulli, SL. Upate on the antibacterial resistance crisis. *Medical Science Monitor.*, 2007, 13 (6), 103-118.

[28] Soupir, M. Occurrence and Movement of Antibiotic Resistant Bacteria and Resistance Genes in Tile-Drained Agricultural Fields Receiving Swine Manure Application. *National Pork Board.*, 2011, 10-119.

[29] Marshall, BM; Levy, SB. Food animals and antimicrobials: impacts on human health. *Clinical Microbiology Reviews.*, 2011, 24(4),718-733.

[30] Kadlec, K; Fessler, AT; Hauschild, T; Schwarz, S. Novel and uncommon antimicrobial resistance genes in livestock-associated methicillin-resistant *Staphylococcus aureus*. *Clin Microbiol Infection.*, 2012, 18(8), 745-755.

[31] Price, LB; Stegger, M; Hasman, H; Aziz, M; Larsen, J; Andersen, PS; et al. *Staphylococcus aureus* CC398: Host Adaptation and Emergence of Methicillin Resistance in Livestock. *mBio.*, 2012, 3(1),1-6.

[32] De Neeling, AJ; Van Den Broek, MJM; Spalburg, EC; Van Santen-Verheuvel, MG; Dam-Deisz, WDC; Boshuizen, HC; et al. High prevalence of methicillin-resistant *Staphylococcus aureus* in pigs. *Vet Microbiol.*, 2007, 122, 366-372.

[33] Lee, JH. Occurrence of methicillin-resistant *Staphylococcus aureus* strains from cattle and chicken, and analyses of their *mecA, mecR1* and *mecI* genes. *Vet Microbiol.*, 2006,113,137-141.

[34] Cuny, C; Friedrich, A; Kozytska, S; Layer, F; Nubel, U; Ohlsen, K; Strommenger, B; Walther, B; Wieler, L; Witte, W. Emergence of methicillin-resistant *Staphylococcus aureus* (MRSA) in different animal species. *Int J Med Microbiol.*, 2010, 300, 109-117.

[35] EFSA (European Food Safety Authority) and ECDC (European Centre for Disease Prevention and Control). The European Union Summary Report on antimicrobial resistance in zoonotic and indicator bacteria from humans, animals and food in 2012. *EFSA J.*, 2014,12(3), 336.

[36] Loeffler, A; Kearns, AM; Ellington, MJ; Smith, LJ; Unt, VE; Lindsay, JA; et al. First isolation of MRSA ST398 from UK animals: a new challenge for infection control teams? *Journal of Hospital Infection.*, 2009, 72(3), 269-71.

[37] Graveland, H; Wagenaar, JA; Bergs, K; Heesterbeek, H; Heederik, D. Persistence of livestock associated MRSA CC398 in humans is dependent on intensity of animal contact. PLoS One, 2011, 6(2).

[38] Paterson, GK; Larsen, J; Harrison, EM; Larsen, AR; Morgan, FJ; Peacock, SJ; et al. First detection of livestock-associated methicillin-resistant *Staphylococcus aureus* CC398 in bulk tank milk in the United Kingdom, January to July 2012. *Eurosurveillance.*, 2012,17,50.

[39] GOV.UK. Livestock-associated MRSA found at a farm in East Anglia. London: GOV.UK. 26 Nov 2013.

[40] Hartley, H; Watson, C; Nugent, P; Beggs, NE. Dickson, Kearns, A. Confirmation of LA-MRSA in pigs in the UK. *Veterinary Record.*, 2014, 175(3),74-5.

[41] Hall, S; Kearns, A. Eckford. Livestock-associated MRSA detected in pigs in Great Britain. *Veterinary Record.*, 2015, 176(6),151-2.

[42] Van Cleef, BA; Verkade, EJ; Wulf, MW; Buiting, AG; Voss, A; Huijsdens, XW; et al. Kluytmans. Prevalence of livestock-associated MRSA in communities with high pig densities in The Netherlands. *PLoS One.*, 2010, 5 (2).

[43] Cuny, C; Abdelbary, MMH; Köck, R; Layer, F; Scheidemann, W; Werner, G; Witte, W. Methicillin-resistant *Staphylococcus aureus* from infectious in horses in Germany are frequent colonizers of veterinarians but rare among MRSA from infections in humans. *One Health.*, 2016, 2,11-17.

[44] Van Rijen, MM; Van Keulen, PH; Kluytmans, JA. Increase in a Dutch hospital of methicillin-resistant *Staphylococcus aureus* related to animal farming. *Clin Infectious Diseases.*, 2008, 46(2), 261-3.

[45] Voss A; Loeffen, F; Bakker, J; Klaassen, C; Wulf, M. Methicillin-resistant *Staphylococcus aureus* in pig farming. *Emerging Inf Dis.*, 2005, 11(12),1965-6.

[46] Denis, O; Suetens, C; Hallin, M; Catry, B; Ramboer, I; Dispas, M. Methicillin-resistant *Staphylococcus aureus* ST398 in swine farm personnel, Belgium. *Emerg Infect Dis.*, 2009, 15 (7),1098-101.

[47] Cuny, C; Nathaus, R; Layer, F; Strommenger, B; Altmann, D; Witte, W. Nasal colonization of humans with methicillin-resistant *Staphylococcus aureus* (MRSA) CC398 with and without exposure to pigs. *PLoS One.*, 2009, 4 (8).

[48] Köck, R; Harlizius, J; Bressan, N; Laerberg, R; Wieler, LH; Witte, et al. 2009. Prevalence and molecular characteristics of methicillin-resistant *Staphylococcus aureus* (MRSA) among pigs on German farms and import of livestock-related MRSA into hospitals. *Euro J Clin Micro Inf Dis.*, 28(11):1375-82.

[49] Bartels, MD; Boye, K; Rhod Larsen, A; Skov, R; Westh, H. Rapid increase of genetically diverse methicillin-resistant *Staphylococcus aureus*, Copenhagen, Denmark. *Emerg Infect Dis.*, 2007, 13, (10),1533-1540.

[50] Wulf, MW; Markestein, A; Van der Linden, FT; Voss, A; Klaassen, C; Verduin CM. First outbreak of methicillin-resistant *Staphylococcus aureus* ST398 in a Dutch hospital, June 2007. *Eurosurveillance.*, 2008, 13(9), 8051.

[51] Ekkelenkamp, MB; Sekkat, M; Carpaij, N; Troelstra, A; Bonten, MJM. Endocarditis due to methicillin-resistant *Staphylococcus aureus* originating from pigs. *Ned Tijdschr Geneeskd.*, 2006, 150(44), 2442-7.

[52] Pan, A; Battisti, A; Zoncada, A; Bernieri, F; Boldini, M; Franco, A; et al. Community-acquired methicillin-resistant *Staphylococcus aureus* ST398 infection, Italy. *Emerging Inf Dis.*, 2009, 15(5), 845-7.
[53] Witte, W; Strommenger, B; Stanek, C; Cuny C. Methicillin-resistant *Staphylococcus aureus* ST398 in humans and animals, Central Europe. *Emerging Inf Dis.*, 2007, 13(2), 255-8.
[54] Dutch Working Party on Antibiotic Policy (SWAB). Consumption of antimicrobial agents and antimicrobial resistance among medically important bacteria in the Netherlands, 2009. Amsterdam: SWAB.
[55] Welinder-Olsson, C; Floren-Johansson, K; Larsson, L; Oberg, S; Karlsson, L; Ahren, C. Infection with Panton-Valentine leukocidin-positive methicillin-resistant *Staphylococcus aureus* t034. *Emerging Inf Dis.*, 2008, 14(8),1271-2.
[56] Kehrenberg, C; Cuny, C; Strommenger, B; Schwarz, S; Witte, W. Methicillin-resistant and -susceptible *Staphylococcus aureus* strains of clonal lineages ST398 and ST9 from swine carry the multidrug resistance gene *cfr*. *J Antimicrobial Chemo.*, 2009, 53(2), 779-81.

In: *Staphylococcus aureus*
Editor: M. L. R. S. Cunha

ISBN: 978-1-63485-959-2
© 2017 Nova Science Publishers, Inc.

*Chapter 4*

# EPIDEMIOLOGY OF HIGHLY ADAPTABLE CLONES: ST398 AND HUMAN DISEASES

*Lígia Maria Abraão, Mariana Fávero Bonesso, Eliane Patrícia Lino Pereira-Franchi and Maria de Lourdes Ribeiro de Souza da Cunha*[*]
Department of Microbiology and Immunology, Botucatu Institute of Biosciences, UNESP - Univ Estadual Paulista. Botucatu,
São Paulo State, Brazil

## ABSTRACT

*Staphylococcus aureus* still remains as one of the most important pathogens widely disseminated among both hospitals and community settings. Interestingly, recent reports have shown that some *S. aureus* strains are highly adaptable and can jump from humans to animals and to humans again after regaining new resistance and virulence factors. Here we present an epidemiological overview of those strains focusing mainly on ST398, since it is becoming an important infectious agent among humans. Noteworthy, ST398 was considered an important livestock-associated pathogen that could be transmitted to humans and only recently emerged in humans related infections highly virulent. Since *S. aureus* is widely disseminated, other clonal complexes are rising and adapting fast. Furthermore, we will highlight the main epidemiology

---

[*] Corresponding author: cunhamlr@ibb.unesp.br

behind this tricky pathogen and pose an important question: is it molecular epidemiology enough to protect us from *S. aureus* future dissemination?

## INTRODUCTION

*Staphylococcus aureus* is a ubiquitous pathogen responsible for causing a wide range of infections related to the Health System. In addition to the arsenal of virulence factors that this microorganism hosts, the emergence of increasingly resistant strains is a major therapeutic and epidemiological challenge as well as a public health problem. According to data previously described, our understanding of the ecological niches and genetic diversity of Methicillin-resistant *Staphylococcus aureus* (MRSA) has changed dramatically since the turn of the millennium. Before that, the reports referred to MRSA mainly situated in hospitals (hospital-acquired MRSA [HA-MRSA]). However, in the 1990s, new strains of MRSA in individuals with no history of contact with health care services were described. These were then named community-acquired *S. aureus* (CA-MRSA) [1, 2, 3].

A decade later, a third type of MRSA was identified. As it is usually related to individuals who work with animals, it is called livestock-associated MRSA (LA-MRSA). This type has stood out because of its emergence in both hospital and community environments, and also for its peculiarities that differentiate them from the other MRSA. Currently, the use of molecular tools allows tracing the genetic characteristics and accessing factors that promote the high adaptability of certain strains and the success of their prevalence. Among the livestock-associated strains, those belonging to clonal complex 398 (CC398) stand out. They are resistant to digestion with *SmaI* enzyme, which is employed in typing techniques by Pulsed-field Gel Electrophoresis (PFGE), and they do not carry some toxin genes typically found in isolates of animal and human origin [2].

Methicillin-resistant *S. aureus* CC398 was first detected in meat animals such as pigs, and it quickly emerged in humans as cause of major infections that are frequently associated with contact with animals. However, methicillin-susceptible *Staphylococcus aureus* (MSSA) CC398 infections not associated with contact with animals cast doubt on the origin of this clone. Thus, the complete genome of 89 samples of *S. aureus* CC398 from human and animal samples (LA-MRSA) from 19 countries was sequenced in order to determine the origin of this clone. The results strongly suggest that the LA-MRSA

CC398 had an initial origin in humans with MSSA, adapted rapidly in animals and acquired resistance to both methicillin and tetracycline, and then were transmitted to humans again. The use of cephalosporin antibiotics in meat animals in the United States and Europe favored the selection of MRSA CC398 [4].

MRSA sequence type (ST) 398 (MRSA ST398) usually lacks the virulence determinants typically found in HA-MRSA and CA-MRSA. Most MRSA ST398 isolates analyzed did not present Leukocidin Panton-Valentine (PVL) encoding genes, staphylococcal enterotoxins (SE), exfoliative toxins (ET), or toxic shock syndrome toxin (TSST). However, most MRSA ST398 isolates carry hemolysin-encoding genes [5].

## EMERGENCE OF *S. AUREUS* ST398 STRAINS IN HOSPITALS

The isolation of ST398 in hospitals is worrying. In 2011, Brunel and colleagues [6] isolated mostly CC398 strains in a surveillance conducted in the ICU by isolating these samples in patients, staff and the environment. The isolation of this strain in the environment suggests its important role as a reservoir of important pathogens.

Hospital infections by CC398 strains have been frequently reported. Although they were not believed to be easily transmitted between humans, reports of hospital transmission of MRSA CC398 have recently demonstrated that its power of spread and infection is much higher than previously thought. The study suggests that the transmission occurred between asymptomatic carriers in two institutions in Denmark resulting in two fatal infections, which suggests a high pathogenicity and a high capacity of transmission between humans [7].

In China, five MRSA ST398 PVL-positive and resistant to multiple antibiotics were isolated from hospitalized elderly patients with lung and wound infections. All patients recovered after the antibiotic treatment despite the type of infection they had [8]. Two ST398 isolates from skin and soft tissue infections in patients in China were also PVL-positive and one isolate was MRSA-SCC*mec* II, but the other strain was HA-MSSA from a renal transplant patient [9]. PVL gene is unusual among strains from this clonal complex, which is concerning because these strains carry other virulence factors and have become extremely pathogenic to humans.

In Belgium, the frequency of ST398 isolates remained low, less than 2% with its emergence in 2008 and having an unusual resistance pattern even for

MSSA [10]. Both MSSA and MRSA ST398 can cause severe infections as reported in other parts of Europe, North America and Latin America. In New York, cases related to CC398 include recurrent skin infection in multiple body parts (1), genital infection (1), and bloodstream infection (one patient had lung abscess) (4). All samples were MRSA SCC*mec* V spa typing t011, t034, t571. In New Zealand, 9 MRSA isolates from wound swab (6), sputum (1), and screening swab (2) were resistant to beta lactam and tetracycline, two samples resistant to erythromycin and one of them was resistant to clindamycin, as well. Two samples were positive for PVL gene (spA t034), and *blaZ* gene was present in 7 samples. All of them had a variety of biofilm formation protein. Bloodstream infections were reported in France in four different institutions with non-identified mode of transmission [11]. In a study performed in China between 2005 and 2010 in a medical hospital, ST7 and ST398 were the most common isolates in blood samples [12].

Pneumonia cases caused by ST398 can be severe and fatal. A 14 year-old healthy girl developed lethal community-acquired necrotizing pneumonia by MSSA ST398, PVL positive, spa typing t571 [13]. A newborn developed pneumonia by MRSA ST398 acquired from his parents [14]. In Italy, MRSA ST398 was isolated from patients with ventilator-associated pneumonia (VAP). Such strain carried SCC*mec* type IV and was negative for PVL [15]. Seven cases of VAP caused by the ST398 SCC*mec* V were reported in 3 different locations in Germany [16].

Pneumonia caused by MSSA ST398 strains can lead to death as reported in a study conducted in Brazil. Three out of four patients who developed pneumonia died in an ICU and the strains showed a high production of alfa-hemolysin and phenol-soluble modulins (PSMs) alfa-3, suggesting a high virulence profile of those strains [17-18].

Other reports of MSSA ST398 strains isolated from patients hospitalized in Brazil demonstrate the ability of this strain to develop resistance mediated by the *crf* gene [19]. Before this publication, the only report of MRSA strains ST398 in Brazil was of their isolation from samples of bovine mastitis carrying SCC*mec* type V t001[20]. ST398 strains were also found in individuals who had pressure ulcers, lived in the community in Brazil, and had not been hospitalized before [21].

A study which found the transmission capacity of MRSA ST398 between humans in a hospital concluded that this strain is 72% less likely to be transmitted between humans than other strains [22].

## SPREAD OF ST398 *S. AUREUS* STRAINS IN ISOLATES OF COMMUNITY ORIGIN WITH OR WITHOUT EXPOSURE TO LIVESTOCK

Genetic and epidemiological evidence shows that MRSA and MSSA differentiate into two distinct lineages [23]. While MRSA ST398 is more associated with exposure to livestock [24, 25, 26, 27, 28, 31, 32] and is rarely found if not by immediate animal contact, the MSSA ST398 is easily transmitted within the community [23, 29, 30, 31, 32].

The CC398 represents a distinct subgroup of MRSA mostly characterized by ST398, ST752, ST291, or ST753 [33-34] harboring the SCC*mec* types V or IV, accessory gene regulator (*agr*) type I and spas t011, t034, t108, t571, t1451, t2011, 2510, and has already been reported in Europe, North America, and Asia [24, 26, 27, 30, 32, 35, 36]. Several studies have reported the occurrence of MRSA ST398 colonization and/or infection related to direct or indirect contact with animals. Most of these studies were performed either in the countryside or in communities with high density of livestock [24, 25, 28]. There are also reports of MRSA ST398 strains isolation in people who work with animals, such as farmers, veterinarians, and their household members [37, 38, 39].

Nearly half of the strains isolated from colonized patients from rural areas in Slovenia were MRSA ST398. Most of them were asymptomatic carriers and one of them was from wound infection. Three different *spa* types were identified: t011, t034, and t108. Both SCC*mec* type V (n = 14) and SCC*mec* type IV (n = 1) were predominant. None of the isolates were positive for PVL, toxic shock syndrome toxin, or leukocidin *Luk*M. Enterotoxin genes (*sek, sei, selo, selu*) were identified in 7 isolates (46.7%). All isolates were tetracycline resistant, and 27% presented resistance to macrolides and lincosamides. Although there are lots of farming activity in this area, there was no epidemiological information regarding animal contact in the patients studied [24].

In two prospective studies, one on MRSA colonization in patients admitted in the hospital and the other one on CA-MRSA infections, 9 out of the 879 nasal swabs examined had MRSA, and five of them belonged to ST398, spas t899(3), t108(1), and t2922(1). No strains were positive for PVL gene. Twenty CA-MRSA isolates were detected: seventeen were from Skin and Soft Tissue Infections (SSTI) and 3 from other infections. An MRSA isolate from otitis external was t899/ST398/PVL. Despite knowing that this region has a high density of livestock, the authors do not know if any of the participants worked or lived in close contact with such animals [40].

Interestingly, most reports show that ST398 human-related infections are caused by MSSA strains, as seen in the most recent report of asymptomatic carriage among convicts in Dallas County Jail [30]. In this study, the female gender and advanced age were the main risk factors for ST398 (t571) carriage. All strains were susceptible to methicillin, resistant to erythromycin, and most of them were also resistant to clindamycin and were negative for PVL genes. According to the same study, ST398 is highly transmitted due to the wide distribution of this strain compared to the other sequence types [30]. This study found nine people in a single cell with MSSA ST398/t571 isolates carriage, which suggests local spread and high transmissibility.

ST398 colonization or infection is not uncommon in people lacking identified livestock-associated risk factors [26, 41]. Moritz et al. [42] reported ST398 colonization in a daycare employee in Iowa, USA. As part of surveillance, nasal and pharyngeal samples were collected from employees and children. One employee was colonized in the nose and throat with MSSA ST398/*t*571. She was 24 years old and had been working at the facility for ≈5 years. She had not been hospitalized in the previous 12 months. She lived alone and she did not have immediate family members who had had contact with animals or who worked in a processing plant.

The MSSA ST398 was the most prevalent isolate from adults with SSTI in Beijing, China. This study did not show any association between livestock contact and ST398 infection. Differently from most studies that have no PVL-positive isolated strains, Zhao et al. [32] found a great number of strains (64.3%) harboring *pvl* gene. Also in China, Jiang et al. [36] studied patients with purulent SSTI from community and isolated one MSSA ST398/t034/PVL. These findings indicate an unrecognized mode of community transmission due to the lack of animal contact [30, 32, 42].

In a study conducted in Finland, MRSA ST398 was isolated in 10 people, and three of them had no direct contact with animals or with one another [43]. Isolation of ST398 t571 was reported in France and in the United States [11, 13, 29, 30, 42].

In a case-control study, all available MSSA specimens were prospectively collected and tested with an ST398-lineage specific polymerase chain reaction (PCR). The results showed that SSTIs were predominant. Being Hispanic and living in the hospital area were factors independently associated with ST398 infections, which suggested that the colonized community served as the source of infections. Unexpectedly, patients with ST398 infections had also been more frequently hospitalized over the 6 months prior to infection, suggesting that ST398 has emerged as both a community- and hospital-associated pathogen [23].

Thirteen participants were found to be colonized with MSSA ST398/t571/PVL in samples collected from humans in northern Manhattan, New York, USA. Four people from the same family were colonized with ST398, but neither infection nor animal contact was confirmed. As northern Manhattan contains a large population that has close ties with the Dominican Republic, a second collection of *S. aureus* isolates was performed from 89 anonymous infection and colonization isolates from the Dominican Republic. Six isolates were identified as MSSA clone ST398, *spa*-type t571 and one isolate was found to be t3625. PFGE analyses showed that the strains from northern Manhattan and from the Dominican Republic were closely related and that they contrasted with the ST398 isolates from Canada [29]. In another study performed in Martinique and the Dominican Republic, almost 10% of MSSA infections (~10%) were caused by ST5 and ST398 isolates [23, 31]. Both studies suggest international transmission of *S. aureus* ST398 strains in Central and North America [23, 29, 31].

In a study in Colombia, 2009, MSSA ST398/t571 was isolated from a woman reporting a 15-day history of fever, dyspnea, and pain in her leg. Four months earlier, she had received a femoro-popliteal vascular prosthetic graft in her left leg. She reported previous contact with chickens and dogs and she lived in a rural area. *S. aureus* was isolated from her blood culture and was susceptible to methicillin, rifampin, and vancomycin, but it was resistant to clindamycin, erythromycin, gentamicin, levofloxacin, minocycline, moxifloxacin, tetracycline, and trimethoprim/sulfamethoxazole [44].

ST398 is naturally pandemic, has a huge reservoir in livestock animals, and seems to be easily transmitted both from humans to animals and from humans to humans. One of the signs of its potential adaptation in humans is indicated by the acquisition of the most important toxin found in CA-MRSA: PVL, which was previously absent in the early reports. CC398 has considerable ability to colonize and consequently cause infections in people living in urban and rural communities and in hospitals, and may or may not be associated with contact with animals. The emergence of ST398 strains highlights the need for more studies in order to clarify its dynamics and transmissibility, as well as the adoption of control measures, especially in areas with high density of livestock.

## EMERGENCE OF STAPHYLOCOCCI CLONAL COMPLEX RELATED WITH THE INFECTION AND COLONIZATION PROCESS

Although the emergence of ST398 is one of the highlights described in various parts of the world, it is possible to notice that other clonal complexes have also been gaining prominence over time. Epidemiological studies show that most MRSA infections refer to a reduced number of clones, such as CC5, CC8, CC22, CC30, and CC45 [45].

On the other hand, MRSA 72 is one of the major and best known clones. This clonal complex is both in the hospital environment and in the community and it is not associated with PVL production, which ensures a greater virulence potential in most clones, such as USA300. Although such clone usually carries the SCC*mec* IV, it has become an important pathogen in hospitals in South Korea. It can cause pneumonia and bone and joint infections. It does not generally produce PVL, but other toxins can replace the absence of such virulence factor, just as the alpha toxins can. This ST is shown to be less virulent than the USA300, which does not interfere with its spreading. According to reports already described, the CC72 has its main virulence factors controlled by the *agr* System. Thus, in cases of bacteremia, it is suggested that a malfunction occurs in the system leading to increased mortality rates in bacteremia caused by this agent [3].

Another predominant strain of MRSA, the LA-MRSA, is the ST9, which is widespread in Asia. This clone, as well as the CC398, is associated with various host animals, such as pigs, calves and poultry. Even though some diseases have already been reported, the ST9 is linked mainly to asymptomatic colonization [46].

ST1 belongs to CC1 and it is a particularly successful strain associated with human infections. It carries the PVL encoding gene, is CA-MRSA PVL positive, and is also known as USA400. It was first reported in a Dutch patient in 2005-2006, then in an Italian patient in 2007 after a trip to the US and Denmark. In the UK, ST1 PVL-negative isolates spa t127 type SCCmec IVa are among the most common CA-MRSA, and are often associated with the injection of drug users and homeless people. In addition, the spa t127 ST1 isolates have been reported as the sixth most prevalent clone both of MRSA and MSSA. Elsewhere in Europe, there are reports of ST1 t127 isolated in animal strains. These, when compared to clones detected in humans, have a similarity of 75%, and the differences seem to be related to SCC*mec*, some virulence genes, and antibiotic resistance markers [47].

CC239 is also among the strains spread worldwide, especially in hospitals [48]. Comparative genomic studies linked to evolutionary analyses show that there are more than 5 MRSA strains in various locations, such as Asia, North America, South America, Europe, and Australia. In China, where ST239 is widely disseminated, the predominant SCC*mec* type III is found in over 50% of MRSA infections. These strains are mainly associated with two types of spa typing, t030 and t037. A phylogenetic analysis of the spa suggests that the t037 is an ancestor of the ST239 spa type. The ST239 type III t037 was the most prevalent subclone in China before 2000. However, this strain has been gradually replaced by ST239 type III t030 [45, 49].

In Brazil, there is an ST239 variant clone, the GV69. This strain was first described in a patient with wound infection admitted to a state hospital for burn patients in Teresina (in the Northeast of the country) in 2006. The cases of ST239 isolates in Brazil are associated with hospital infections and are widely disseminated, multidrug-resistant, and are usually found grouped in the middle of a Brazilian epidemic clone. GV69, as well as other STs already described, shows a natural dysfunction in *agr* system, is a moderate phenotype to biofilm production, and carries genes with hemolytic activity [48].

In the years 2004/2005 in India, a CA-MRSA clone PVL positive was described: the ST772-MRSA-V, colloquially known as Bengal Bay Clone. The spread of Bengal Bay MRSA occurred in several countries, including England, Ireland, Germany (HJ Linde and Regensburg), Norway, Italy, the United Arab Emirates (Abu Dhabi), Saudi Arabia, Hong Kong, Malaysia, Australia, and New Zealand. Many individuals in which the clone was identified had a history of traveling to or having relatives living in some of the mentioned places, which suggests the occurrence of infection in India, Pakistan, and Bangladesh, and also Linde and Regensburg in Germany, which are places where this strain seems to be increasingly more common. According to analyzes performed by Multilocus sequence typing (MLST) *e-burst*, ST772 appears to be related to CC1, differing from such ST in only one allele. However, because of numerous distinctions, their inclusion to the CC1 must be reevaluated [50].

Some studies show that hospital-acquired MRSA isolates have different genetic characteristics and are spread across different geographical regions. Most of the clones seem to have arisen in Europe, such as ST8, ST247, ST239, and ST228, which are clones prevalent in Italy. Multiresistant HA-MRSA strains are characterized by ST111-MRSA-I in Croatia, ST8 MRSA-IV in

France, and ST228 I, II ST5 in Hungary. There is also a wide range of HA-MRSA clones in Asia, where the following clones are predominant: ST6-IV clone t304 in Oman, ST239-MRSA III in Saudi Arabia, ST239-MRSA IV in Iran, ST239-MRSA II in China, India, and Indonesia, ST5- MRSA II in Korea and Japan, and ST30-MRSA IV in Qatar. Among these, ST22 must be highlighted as it is characterized as a global pandemic clone that emerged in England in 1991 and was thus named UK-MRSA-15 [51].

There are few studies addressing the potential impacts of specific *S. aureus* clones and their clinical manifestations and mortality rates. Nevertheless, CC 5, 8, 15, 30 and 45 appear to be the most prevalent clones that usually cause invasive diseases [52].

Clones belonging to CC5 and CC30 have been associated with bacteremia and other hematologic complications. The clonal complex CC5 is a quite common CA-MRSA, which is widespread throughout the world (Shady et al., 2015). ST30 is connected to cases of infective endocarditis. Surprisingly, the first LA-MRSA CC30 was isolated encoding a recognized virulence marker (*lukM*) from fattening pigs in Northern Ireland in 2015 [46].

For over three decades, MRSA has become endemic in Ireland. Interestingly, there were several clonal replacements throughout such period. During the last decade, MRSA ST22, IV SCC*mec* isolates were predominant; they were present in 80% of the recovered samples of patients in Irish hospitals. Currently, it can be seen that between 2006 and 2011, there was the emergence of the rare clonal complex ST779 spa 878. The sequence analysis of the genome of this clone identified an important feature. The ST779 has a new pseudo composition, the element SCC*mec*-SCC-SCCCRISPR, which carries a CRISPR encoding a prokaryotic defense mechanism against foreign DNA. It is still an open question whether this new CC will be able to become one of the most worldwide spread clones. However, it is noteworthy that this new composition element that it harbors can grant advantageous attributes in addition to the resistance to methicillin mechanisms, such as resistance to copper and fusidic acid, and the mechanism of resistance to or immunity against foreign DNA encoded by the CRISPR. Several other ST779 or closely related isolates were previously described, suggesting that this clone was already present in some regions such as Australia, Canada, Germany, Thailand, the United Arab Emirates, and England [53].

The emergence of *S. aureus* strains belonging to highly adaptable STs both in humans and in animals reinforces the need for epidemiological and molecular investigations given the importance of this agent in a wide range of infections. New sequence types have been emerging and increasing their prevalence compared to classical clones as ST8 (USA300) which is highly virulent in humans and is able to adapt in domestic animals like dogs. Thus, surveillance methods and the use of tools that enable the monitoring of the evolution of this strain are highly important in order to invest heavily on measures that ensure the control of *S. aureus* spread in general.

## REFERENCES

[1] Smith, TC; and Shylo; EW. Human Infections with *Staphylococcus aureus* CC398. *Curr Environ Health Rep.*, 2015, 2(1), 41–51.

[2] Groves, MD; Bethany C; Geoffrey, WC; David, J; Stanley, P; Mary, DB; Phil, G; Sam, A; and Darren, JT. Molecular Epidemiology of Methicillin-Resistant *Staphylococcus aureus* Isolated from Australian Veterinarians., 2016, *PLoS One.*, 11 (1), 1–12.

[3] Joo, EJ; Choi, JY; Chung, DR; Song, JH; Ko, KS. Characteristics of the Community-Genotype Sequence Type 72 Methicillin-Resistant *Staphylococcus aureus* Isolates That Underlie Their Persistence in Hospitals. *J Microbiol.*, 2016, 54(6), 445–50.

[4] Price, LB; Stegger, M; Hasman, H; Aziz, M; Larsen, J; Andersen, S; Pearson, T; et al. *Staphylococcus aureus* CC398 : Host Adaptation and Emergence of Methicillin Resistance in Livestock. *mBio.*, 2012, 3(1), 1–7.

[5] Zarfel, G; Krziwanek, K; Johler, S; Hoenigl, M; Leitner, E; Kittinger, C; Masoud, L; Feierl, G; Grisold, AJ. Virulence and Antimicrobial Resistance Genes in Human MRSA ST398 Isolates in Austria. *Epidemiol Infect.*, 2013, 141(4), 888–92.

[6] Brunel, AS; Bañuls, AL; Marchandin, H; Bouzinbi, N; Morquin, D; Jumas-bilak, E; Corne, P. J. Methicillin-sensitive *Staphylococcus aureus* CC398 in intensive care unit, France. *Emerg Infect Dis.*, 2014, 20(9), 1511-5.

[7] Nielsen, RT; Kemp, M; Holm, A; Skov, NM; Detlefsen, M; Hasman, H et al. Fatal Septicemia Linked to Transmission of MRSA Clonal Complex 398 in Hospital and Nursing Home, Denmark. *Emerg Infect Dis.*, 2016, 22 (5), 1–3.

[8] Yu, F; Chen, Z; Liu, C; Zhang, X; Lin, X; Chi, S; Zhou, T; Chen, Z; Chen, X. Prevalence of *Staphylococcus aureus* carrying Panton-Valentine leukocidin genes among isolates from hospitalised patients in China. *Clin Microbiol Infect.*, 2008, 14(4), 381-4.

[9] Yao, D; Fang-yo, Y; Zhi-qiang, Q; Chun, C; Su-su, H, Zeng-qiang, C; Xue-qing, Z. Molecular Characterization of *Staphylococcus aureus* Isolates Causing Skin and Soft Tissue Infections. *BMC Infect Dis.*, 2010, 10(1), 133.

[10] Vandendriessche, S; Hallin, M; Catry, B; Jans, B; Deplano, A; Nonhoff, C; Roisin, S; Struelens, MJ; Denis, O. Previous Healthcare Exposure Is the Main Antecedent for Methicillin-Resistant *Staphylococcus aureus* Carriage on Hospital Admission in Belgium. *Eur J Clin Microbiol Infect Dis.*, 2012, 31(9), 2283-92.

[11] Van Der Mee-Marquet, N; Francois, P; Domelier-Valentin, AS; Coulomb, F;l Decreux, C; Hombrock-Allet, C; Lehiani, O; et al. Emergence of Unusual Bloodstream Infections Associated with Pig-Borne-like *Staphylococcus aureus* ST398 in France. *Clin Infect Dis.*, 2011, 52(1), 152–53.

[12] Song, Y; Du, X; Li, T; Zhu, Y; Li, M. Phenotypic and Molecular Characterization of *Staphylococcus aureus* Recovered from Different Clinical Specimens of Inpatients at a Teaching Hospital in Shanghai between 2005 and 2010. *J Med Microbiol.*, 2013, 62(2), 274–82.

[13] Rasigade, JP; Laurent, F; Vandenesch, F. Lethal Necrotizing Pneumonia Caused by an ST398 *Staphylococcus aureus* Strain. *Emerg Infect Dis.*, 2010, 16(8), 1330.

[14] Hartmeyer, GN; Gahrn-Hansen, B; Skov, RL; Kolmos, HJ. Pig-associated methicillin-resistant *Staphylococcus aureus*: family transmission and severe pneumonia in a newborn. *Scand J Infect Dis.*, 2010, 42(4), 318-20.

[15] Mammina, C; Calà, C; Plano, MRA; Bonura, C; Vella, A; Monastero, R; Palma, DM. Ventilator-Associated Pneumonia and MRSA ST398, Italy. *Emerg Infect Dis.*, 2010, 16(4), 730–31.

[16] Wolfgang, W; Strommenger, B; Stanek, C; Cuny, C. *Staphylococcus aureus* ST398 in Humans and Animals, Central Europe. *Emerg Infect Dis.*, 2007, 13(2), 255–58.

[17] Rebollo-Pérez, J; Ordoñez-Tapia, C; Herazo-Herazo, C; Reyes-Ramos, N. Nasal Carriage of Panton Valentine Leukocidin-Positive Methicillin-Resistant *Staphylococcus aureus* in Healthy Preschool Children. *Rev. salud pública.*, 2011, 13(5), 824–32.

[18]  Bonesso, MF; Yeh, AJ; Villaruz, AE; Joo, HS; McCausland, J; Fortaleza, CM; Cavalcante, RS; Sobrinho, MT; Ronchi, CF; Cheung, GY; Cunha, ML; Otto, M. Key Role of α-Toxin in Fatal Pneumonia Caused by *Staphylococcus aureus* Sequence Type 398. *Am J Respir Crit Care Med*, 2016, 193(2), 217-20

[19]  Gales, AC; Lalitagauri, MD; souza, AG; Pignatari, ACC; Mendes, RE. MSSA ST398/t034 Carrying a Plasmid-Mediated *Cfr* and *Erm*(B) in Brazil. *J Antimicrob Chemother.*, 2015, 70(1), 303–5.

[20]  Silva, NCC; Guimarães, FF; Manzi, MP; Junior, AF; Gimenez-Sanz, E; Gimenez, P; Langoni, H; Rall, VLM; Torres, C. Methicillin-Resistant *Staphylococcus aureus* of Lineage ST398 as Cause of Mastitis in Cows. *Lett Appl Microbiol.*, 2014, 59(6), 665–69.

[21]  Franch, EPLP. Epidemiologia molecular e estudo dos fatores de virulência de *Staphylococcus aureus* resistentes à oxacilina isolados de feridas em pacientes atendidos em unidades básicas de saúde da cidade de Botucatu. Tese (doutorado) Universidade Estadual Paulista "Júlio de Mesquita Filho" (UNESP). Botucatu-SP.

[22]  Wassenberg, MWM; Bootsma, MCJ; Troelstra, A; Kluytmans, JAJW; Bonten, MJM. Transmissibility of Livestock-Associated Methicillin-Resistant *Staphylococcus aureus* (ST398) in Dutch Hospitals. *Clin Microbiol Infect.*, 2010,17(2), 316–19.

[23]  Uhlemann, AC; Hafer, C; Miko, BA; Sowash, MG; Sullivan, SB; Shu, Q; Lowy, FD. Emergence of Sequence Type 398 as a Community- and Healthcare- Associated Methicillin-Susceptible *Staphylococcus aureus* in Northern Manhattan. *Clin Infect Dis.*, 2013, 57(5), 700-703.

[24]  Dermota, U; Košnik, IG; Müller-premru, M; Zajc, U; Golob, M; Rupnik, M. Molecular Characterization of Methicillin- Resistant *Staphylococcus aureus*, ST398 (LA-MRSA), from Human Samples. *Slov Vet Res.*, 2015, 52 (3), 155-60.

[25]  Graveland, H; Wagenaar, JA; Bergs, K; Heesterbeek, H; Heederik, D. Persistence of Livestock Associated MRSA CC398 in Humans Is Dependent on Intensity of Animal Contact. *PLoS ONE.*, 2011, 6(2), e16830.

[26]  Wulf, MWH; Markestein, A; Van Der Linden, FT; Voss, A; Klaassen, C; Verduin, CM. First outbreak of methicillin-resistant *Staphylococcus aureus* ST398 in a Dutch hospital, June 2007. *Euro Surveill.*, 2008,13, 8051.

[27] Denis, O; Suetens, C; Hallin, M; Catry, B; Ramboer, I; Dispas, M; Willems, G; Gordts, B; Butaye, P; Struelens, MJ. Methicillin-Resistant *Staphylococcus aureus* ST398 in Swine Farm Personnel, Belgium. *Emerg Infect Dis.*, 2009, 15(7), 1098-1101.

[28] Angelo, P; Battisti, A; Zoncada, A; Bernieri, F; Boldini, M; Franco, A; Giorgi, M; Iurescia, M; Lorenzotti, L; Martinotti, M; Monaci, M; Pantosti, AA. Communityacquired MethicillinResistant *Staphylococcus aureus* ST398 Infection, Italy. *Emerg Infect Dis.*, 2009, 132(1-2), 145–59.

[29] Bhat, M; Dumortier, C; Taylor, BS; Miller, M; Vasquez, G; Yunen, J; Brudney, K; et al. *Staphylococcus aureus* ST398, New York City and Dominican Republic. *Emerg Infect Dis.*, 2009, 15(2), 285-287.

[30] Michael, D; Siegel, J; Lowy, FD; Zychowski, D; Taylor, A; Lee, CJ; Boyle-Vavra, S; Daum, RS. Asymptomatic Carriage of Sequence Type 398, Spa Type t571 Methicillin-Susceptible *Staphylococcus aureus* in an Urban Jail: A Newly Emerging, Transmissible Pathogenic Strain. *J Clin Microbiol.*, 2013, 51(7), 2443-7.

[31] Ulemann, AC; Dumortier, C; Hafer, C; Taylor, BS; Sanchez, J; Rodrigues-Taveras, C; Leon, P; Rojas, R; Olive, C; Lowy, FD. Molecular Characterization of *Staphylococcus aureus* from Outpatients in the Caribean Reveals the Presence of Pandemic Clones. *Eur J Clin Microbiol Infect Dis.*, 2012, 4(164), 505–11.

[32] Zhao, C; Liu, Y; Zhao, M; Liu,Y; Yu, Y; Chen, H; Sun, Q; et al. Characterization of Community Acquired *Staphylococcus aureus* Associated with Skin and Soft Tissue Infection in Beijing: High Prevalence of PVL + ST398. *PLoS ONE.*, 7(6), e38577.

[33] Loo, IV; Huijsdens, X; Tiemersma, E; De Neeling, A. Emergence of Methicillin-Resistant *Staphylococcus aureus* of Animal Origin in Humans. *Emerg Infect Dis.*, 2007, 13, 1834–1839.

[34] Mediavilla, JR; Chen, L; Uhlemann, AC; Hanson, BM; Rosenthal, M; Stanak, K; Koll, B; et al. Methicillin-Susceptible *Staphylococcus aureus* ST398, New York and New Jersey, USA. *Emerg Infect Dis.*, 2012, 18(4), 700–702.

[35] Tavares, A; Miragaia, M; Rolo, J; Coelho, C; Lencastre, H. High Prevalence of Hospital-Associated Methicillin-Resistant *Staphylococcus aureus* in the Community in Portugal: Evidence for the Blurring of Community – Hospital Boundaries. *Eur J Clin Microbiol Infect Dis.*, 2013, 32(10), 1269-83.

[36] Jiang, W; Zhou, Z; Zhang, K; Yu, Y. Epidemiological investigation of community-acquired *Staphylococcus aureus* infection. *Genet Mol Res.*, 12 (4), 6923-6930.

[37] Lozano, C; Marí, A; Aspiroz, C; Gómez-sanz, E; Ceballos, S; Barcenilla, F; Jover-sáenz, A; Torres, C; Fortu, B. Nasal Carriage of Coagulase Positive Staphylococci in Patients of a Primary-Healthcare-Center : Genetic Lineages and Resistance and Virulence Genes. *Enferm Infecc Microbiol Clin.*, 2015, 33(6), 391–396.

[38] Velasco, V; Buyukcangaz, E; Sherwood, JS; Stepan, RM; Koslofsky, RJ; Logue, CM. Characterization of *Staphylococcus ureus* from Humans and a Comparison with İsolates of Animal Origin, in North Dakota, United States. *Plos One.*, 2015, 10(10), e0140497.

[39] Garcia-graells, C; Antoine, J; Larsen, J; Catry, B; Skov, R; Denis, O. Livestock Veterinarians at High Risk of Acquiring Methicillin-Resistant *Staphylococcus aureus* ST398. *Epidemiol. Infect.*, 2012, 140(03), 383–89.

[40] Monaco, M; Pedroni, P; Sanchini, A; Bonomini, A; Indelicato, A; Pantosti, AL. Livestock-Associated Methicillin-Resistant *Staphylococcus aureus* Responsible for Human Colonization and Infection in an Area of Italy with High Density of Pig Farming. *BMC Infect Dis.*, 2013, 13(1), 258.

[41] Golding, GR; Bryden, L; Levett, PN; McDonald, RR: Wong, A; Wylie, J; Graham, MR; et al. Livestock-Associated Methicillin-Resistant *Staphylococcus aureus* Sequence Type 398 in Humans, Canada. *Emerg Infect Dis.*, 2010, 16(4), 587–94.

[42] Moritz, ED; Smith, TS. Livestock- Associated *Staphylococcus aureus* in Childcare Worker. *Emerg Infect Dis.*, 2011, 43(9), 1143–51.

[43] Salmenlinna, S; Lyytikäinen, O; Vainio, A; Myllyniemi, AL; Raulo, S; Kanerva, M; Rantala, M; Thomson, K. Human Cases of 2010. Human Cases of Methicillin-Resistant *Staphylococcus aureus* CC398, Finland. *Emerg Infect Dis.*, 2010,16(10), 1626-1629.

[44] Jiménez, JN; Vélez, LA; Mediavilla, JR; Ocampo, AM; Vanegas, JM; Rodríguez, EA; Kreiswirth, BN; Correa, MM. Livestock- Associated Methicillin- Susceptible *Staphylococcus aureus* ST398 Infection in Woman, Colombia. *Emerg Infect Dis.*, 2011, 17(10), 1970–71.

[45] Shang, W; Hu, Q; Yuan, W; Cheng, H; Yang, J; Hu, Z; Yuan, J; et al. Comparative Fitness and Determinants for the Characteristic Drug Resistance of ST239-MRSAIII-t030 and ST239-MRSA-III-t037 Strains Isolated in China. *Microb Drug Resist.*, 2015, 22(3), 185-92.

[46] Lahuerta-marin, A; Guelbenzu-gonzalo, M; Pichon, B; Allen, A; Doumith, M; Lavery, JF; Watson, C; Teale, CJ; Kearns, AM. First Report of lukM - First report of lukM-positive livestock-associated methicillin-resistant Staphylococcus aureus CC30 from fattening pigs in Northern Ireland. *Vet Microbiol.*, 2016, 15,(182), 131-4.

[47] Alba, P; Feltrin, F; Cordaro, G; Porrero, MC; Kraushaar, B; Argudín, MA Nykäsenoja, S; et al. Livestock-Associated Methicillin Resistant and Methicillin Susceptible *Staphylococcus aureus* Sequence Type (CC)1 in European Farmed Animals: High Genetic Relatedness of Isolates from Italian Cattle Herds and Humans. *PLoS ONE* 2015., 10(8), 1–10.

[48] Botelho, AMN; Costa, MOC; Beltrame, CO; Ferreira, FA; Côrtes, MF; Bandeira, PT; Lima, NCB; et al. Complete Genome Sequence of an Agr-Dysfunctional Variant of the ST239 Lineage of the Methicillin-Resistant *Staphylococcus aureus* Strain GV69 from Brazil. *Stand Genomic Sci.,2016*, 11(1), 34.

[49] Qingzhong, L; Han, L; Li, B; Sun, J; and Ni, Y. Virulence Characteristic and MLST-Agr Genetic Background of High-Level Mupirocin-Resistant, MRSA Isolates from Shanghai and Wenzhou, China. *PloS One.*, 2012, 7(5), e37005.

[50] Monecke, S; Coombs, GW; Pearson, J; Hotzel, H; Slickers, P; Ehricht, R. A Clonal Complex 12 Methicillin-Resistant *Staphylococcus aureus*. *Antimicrob Agents Chemother.*, 2015, 59(11), 7142–44.

[51] Mehdi, G; Goudarzi, H; Figueiredo, AMS; Udo, EE; Fazeli, M; Asadzadeh, M; Seyedjavadi, SS. Molecular Characterization of Methicillin Resistant *Staphylococcus aureus* Strains Isolated from Intensive Care Units in Iran: ST22-SCCmec IV/t790 Emerges as the Major Clone. *Plos One.*, 2016, 11(5), e0155529.

[52] Blomfeldt, A., A. N. Eskesen, H. V. Aamot, T. M. Leegaard, and J. V. Bjrnholt. Population-Based Epidemiology of *Staphylococcus aureus* Bloodstream Infection: Clonal Complex 30 Genotype Is Associated with Mortality. *Eur J Clin Microbiol Infect Dis.*, 2016, 35(5), 803–13.

[53] Kinnevey, P M; Shore, AC; Brennan, GI; Sullivan, DJ; Ehricht, R; Monecke, S; Slickers, P; Coleman, DC. Emergence of Sequence Type 779 Methicillin-Resistant *Staphylococcus aureus* Harboring a Novel Pseudo Staphylococcal Cassette Chromosome Mec (SCCmec)-SCC-SCCCRISPR Composite Element in Irish Hospitals. *Antimicrob Agents Chemother.*, 2013, 57(1), 524–31.

In: *Staphylococcus aureus*
Editor: M. L. R. S. Cunha

ISBN: 978-1-63485-959-2
© 2017 Nova Science Publishers, Inc.

*Chapter 5*

# *STAPHYLOCOCCUS* SPP. IN BLOODSTREAM INFECTIONS

*Aydir Cecília Marinho Monteiro* and
*Maria de Lourdes Ribeiro de Souza da Cunha*[*]
Department of Microbiology and Immunology, Botucatu Institute of
Biosciences, UNESP - Univ Estadual Paulista. Botucatu,
São Paulo State, Brazil

## ABSTRACT

Bloodstream infections (BSIs) have gained importance due to the increase in their incidence in recent years. BSIs increase the length of hospital stay, the costs associated and the patients' morbidity and mortality rates. Early diagnosis, in addition to the identification of the microorganism and its sensitivity to antimicrobial agents, has great diagnostic and prognostic importance. Several microorganisms are isolated in the bloodstream; however, multicenter studies have found *Staphylococcus aureus* and coagulase-negative staphylococci (CoNS) as the major etiological agents of bloodstream infections in recent decades. The examination of blood cultures is the primary means of etiological diagnosis available in clinical practice, although the step of identifying these microorganisms by conventional methods is a lengthy process. Automation is a fast and reliable option from studies that show improved performance of automated equipment, but such equipment is still not able

---

[*] Corresponding author: cunhamlr@ibb.unesp.br

to accurately identify the different species of CoNS because of either the slow metabolism of sugars or the variable expressions of the phenotypic traits of some of these species. The use of molecular biology techniques for bacterial identification in such cases is a solution because the results obtained are fast, accurate and sensitive, and also because the identifications performed with DNA extracted directly from blood cultures decrease the duration of the identification process significantly. This chapter aims at discussing the prevalence of *Staphylococcus aureus* and CoNS in BSIs by highlighting the automation techniques and molecular biology techniques as alternatives for the fast and accurate identification of *Staphylococcus* spp., which allows the quick start of a specific treatment.

## INTRODUCTION

Bloodstream infection (BSI) is defined as the presence of viable microorganisms circulating in the blood confirmed laboratorial [1]. These microorganisms are either from the patient's microbiota or resulting from contamination due to improper handling of such patient by health professionals [2].

The BSIs have showed an increase in their incidence since the 1991 survey conducted by the American agency National Nosocomial Infections Surveillance (NNIS), the current National Healthcare Safety Network (NHSN). This increase is justified by the progress in health care and by the use of invasive devices, particularly the intravenous catheter, in the treatment and monitoring of critically ill patients in intensive care units (ICU) [3-5].

Sepsis, the clinical condition due to the worsening of the BSI, is defined as the systemic inflammatory response to the infectious agent. It refers to the circulatory system and results from complex interactions between the patient's immune system and the infecting microorganism, which multiplies at a rate that exceeds its removal from the body [6]. It is a clinical syndrome characterized by fever, chills, malaise, tachycardia, hyperventilation, toxicity, and prostration. Its symptoms are produced by microbial toxins and/or cytokines produced by inflammatory cells [7]. Such infection is considered to be a public health problem because it increases the morbidity and mortality of patients, their hospital stay, and the costs of the treatment [8]. In addition, it is the main cause of mortality of patients in critical condition [9] with rates ranging from 20% to 50% [10]. Sepsis is known as the second cause of noncoronary death in ICUs in the United States and the main cause in Latin

American countries [11], and in Brazil it was considered to be the biggest public health problem in the Brazilian Sepsis Epidemiological Study (BASES study) [12]. The Center for Disease Control (CDC) noted that cases of sepsis in the United States increased from 621,000 in 2000 to 1,141,000 in 2008 [13], and between the years 2003 and 2007 there was an increase in cases of sepsis from 415,000 to 700,000 per year, which raised the associated costs from US$15.4 billion to US$24.3 billion in such period [14]. It is estimated that 17 million cases occur worldwide annually, and 600,000 of them occur in Brazil alone [11].

## PREVALENCE OF *STAPHYLOCOCCUS AUREUS* AND CONS IN BSIS

Numerous microorganisms are isolated from the bloodstream, and among the bacteria, Gram-negative bacilli have higher associated mortality compared to Gram-positive cocci, but they have become less frequent in bloodstream infections since the 1990s [15, 16]. The National Healthcare Safety Network (NHSN) conducted a data survey between 2006 and 2007, and it pointed coagulase-negative *Staphylococcus* (CoNS) as the main causative agents of infections [17]. This fact was repeated in the data presented in 2013 on the survey conducted between 2009 and 2010 [18].

Data from the Surveillance and Control of Pathogens of Epidemiological Importance (SCOPE) in the US relating to a period of seven years from March 1995 to September 2002 indicated that the Gram-positive cocci were the main bloodstream infection agents (65%) and the CoNS were the most frequent of them (31%) followed by *Staphylococcus aureus* (20%)[4]. *Staphylococcus aureus* (14%) and CoNS (12.6%) were revealed as the most isolated microorganisms according to the Brazilian data collected between June 2007 and March 2010 from a multicenter study using the same methodology of the American SCOPE program - the Brazilian SCOPE - aiming at studying the epidemiology and microbiology of nosocomial bloodstream infections of patients from 16 Brazilian hospitals of various sizes and different regions [19]. Data from the Hospital Infection Surveillance System of São Paulo State, Epidemiological Surveillance Center (ESC), also reported the CoNS as the agents most associated with bloodstream infection in 2010. *Staphylococcus epidermidis* and other CoNS were the most predominant (30.1%) followed by *Staphylococcus aureus* (16.6%) [20]. The prevalence of CoNS was repeated in the results showed in studies conducted in Asian and South American countries between 2006 and 2013 [8, 21, 22, 23].

The *Staphylococcus* genus consists of 52 species [24] classified into two groups according to the production capacity of the coagulase enzyme. The first group, known as coagulase positive staphylococci, has *S. aureus* as its main representative [25]. In the second group, known as coagulase-negative staphylococci (CoNS), the main species involved in human infections are *S. epidermidis*, *S. haemolyticus*, *S. saprophyticus*, *S. cohnii*, *S. xylosus*, *S. capitis*, *S. warneri*, *S. hominis*, *S. simulans*, and *S. lugdunensis* [26, 27].

The CoNs bacteria are part of the human microbiota, that is, they are natural inhabitants of the skin and mucous membranes of humans and live symbiotically with their host. In cases of skin barrier trauma, inoculation using needles, and implantation of medical devices (catheters, prostheses, and others), these microorganisms acquire pathogenic potential and can cause serious infections. They are the most frequently isolated microorganisms in clinical devices [28, 29].

The CoNS were previously considered non-pathogenic, and nowadays they are involved in urinary tract infections, endocarditis, and peritoneal dialysis-associated peritonitis both in immunocompromised hosts and in healthy subjects [30]. In the last three decades, they have been associated with infections in immunosuppressed patients, premature infants, and patients with implants and prostheses. Currently, they are mainly known as essentially opportunistic microorganisms which are prevalent in a number of organic situations as they lead to severe infections [31, 32]. In the hospital setting, the CoNS are the main causes of BSI mostly in patients kept in ICUs [28].

Studies are unanimous in reporting the *S. epidermidis* as the most common species of CoNS isolates in infections [33, 34, 35] known to cause sepsis and infections arising from implanting prostheses and catheters and from peritonitis [36]. *S. haemolyticus*, part of the microbiota of the human skin, can cause meningitis, endocarditis, peritonitis, and sepsis [37]. This is the second species of CoNS most isolated in blood cultures [37, 38, 39, 40, 41]. *S. hominis*, a commensal microorganism of the human skin, is a potential cause of endocarditis and catheter-related infections [42]. It is an opportunistic pathogen associated with bacteremia and eye infections, endocarditis, peritonitis, osteomyelitis, and infections with other microorganisms [31, 44, 45, 46].The species *S. capitis*, part of the normal microbiota of the scalp, face, neck and ears [47] can cause serious infections in native valves in immunocompromised patients with valvular heart diseases [48] besides being related to urinary tract infections [49] and bacteremia resulting from using catheters [50].

## DIAGNOSTIC LABORATORY

Confirming the presence of microorganisms present in blood cultures is among the most important roles of the clinical microbiology laboratory [51] because the examination of blood culture - the gold standard in the diagnosis of sepsis - is able to elucidate the etiology and lead to the appropriate antibiotic treatment in order to improve the prognosis of patients in sepsis and, therefore, reduce the morbidity and mortality [52, 53]. Early diagnosis of sepsis followed by the appropriate treatment improves the patient's prognosis [54]. The rapid identification of the microorganism causing sepsis is crucial for an accurate therapeutic approach with significant clinical benefits [55] as the appropriate antimicrobial therapy with an early start is essential in determining the prognosis and survival of the patient with bloodstream infection [56, 57]. This importance is evident in the cases of patients receiving antibiotic therapy appropriate to the sensitivity profile of the infectious agent isolated in culture. They had lower mortality than the patients who received inadequate antibiotic therapy, and such treatment was later adjusted with the diagnosis obtained from the culture [7]. Early diagnosis followed by the appropriate treatment improves the prognosis of a septic patient [58-60]). Every hour delay in administering the correct antibiotic is associated with an average reduction of 8% in the survival rate of septic shock [61]. Another important factor associated with early appropriate treatment is the decrease in the use of empirical antibiotic therapy that reduces the risk of resistant microorganisms emerging within the hospital environment[62-64].

Presently, technological advances able to provide a fast and reliable microbial identification for most pathogens involved in infectious diseases are seen as a way to bring clinical and financial benefits [65]. The work of the clinical microbiology laboratory in the detection and identification of BSI-causing microorganism is fundamental [65, 66] and the examination of blood culture is one of the main roles of such type of laboratory [51]. The blood culture tests in most clinical microbiology laboratories are automated, which considerably reduced the time spent on the testing, but the steps following the growth of microorganisms in the blood culture take from 48 to 72 hours. These steps are the isolation, identification, and antimicrobial susceptibility testing (AST) of the microorganisms. The delay occurs because the identification of the microorganism is performed through conventional phenotypic methods based on Gram staining, analysis of morphological structures, nutritional requirements for growth, and biochemical reactions presented by the microorganism [67]. Although conventional phenotypic methods are relatively inexpensive and allow the identification of the most common microorganisms, certain groups of bacteria are difficult to identify and often require specific equipment [68]. This delay in the processes subsequent to the positive blood culture calls for the development of faster and more efficient methods for the identification of isolated microorganisms and their AST, especially when it comes to the inherent urgency in cases of sepsis [69]. A large number of commercial blood culture systems are available. They consist of a conventional blood culture broth, lysis-centrifugation system, and automated systems [70]. Automation in clinical microbiology occurred as a response to the increasing number of clinical isolates processed in routine microbiology laboratories and it was facilitated by the interface between the computer systems of laboratories and the hospitals [71]. In such scenario, several automated systems have been produced for the identification of microorganisms and production of AST. The species identification is based on automatic interpretation of the results of biochemical tests or from microdilution trays after overnight incubation and determination of the growth through photometry [72-74].

Satisfactory performance of automated methodologies with acceptable and accurate results has been demonstrated in recent decades in the routine of clinical microbiology laboratories [75]. In order to decrease the time spent to identify microorganisms, a variety of automated systems for their identification have been developed based on the automatic interpretation of the results of biochemical testing and on the determination of the growth of microorganisms by photometry [72, 73, 76, 77]. However, a recurring fact observed with such equipment was the failure to identify the Gram-positive cocci, especially among the species of coagulase-negative *Staphylococcus* [78-80]. These rather unreliable results are due to the inability of automated systems to detect the variable expression of the phenotypic characteristics of such bacteria [7] because of the slow metabolism of certain species which leads to an ambiguous result in their identification [81].

Devices that perform the identification of microorganisms by mass spectrometry have recently been developed. This analytical technique is known as MALDI-TOF (Matrix Assisted Laser Desorption Ionization Time-of-Flight) and it provides the elemental composition of the sample. It consists of the ionization of chemical components to create charged molecules and to measure its mass relative to the mass load creating molecular signatures that can be used for rapid bacterial identification from isolated colonies.The use of mass spectrometry for bacterial identification presents good benefit cost and has been specially developed for clinical microbiology laboratories with high sample volume [82]. The routine use of mass spectrometry in clinical microbiology laboratories is reported, but its performance and its accuracy are not yet fully understood. Its use in the identification of microorganisms isolated directly from blood culture bottles did not show satisfactory results in studies with a large number of samples either [83-85] possibly due to the interference of blood components with the measurementof MALDI-TOF, which demonstrates the need for protocols with several centrifugations and washings [86].

The molecular biological methods for the identification of microorganisms are a viable alternative for such type of identification for their rapidity, accuracy, and sensitivity in the results obtained [69]. Molecular biology techniques have become easier and cheaper, and their use in the detection and identification of microorganisms in clinical analysis routines occurs by using signal amplification methods, polymerase chain reaction (PCR) which evolved and became real-time PCR, and the use of genetic typing techniques that demonstrate the relationship between microorganisms and inform about the transmission of infectious diseases [87].

PCR is a DNA replication technique with the amplification of a specific region of the genome which can be used to obtain useful information for the diagnosis of patients with infections [88]. These PCR reactions and the sequencing of DNA regions of the 16S rRNA gene are a solution for the identification to the species level or they are a supplement to the conventional phenotypic methods for the species that are difficult to be identified conventionally [89, 90]. In order to reduce the time spent on the identification of microorganisms and to make the DNA extraction directly from microorganisms grown in blood culture possible, different extraction techniques have been developed and improved so as to allow the identification of microorganisms by using molecular biology techniques - especially the PCR reactions - to be performed quickly and effectively, and, thus, reduce the misidentification that routinely occurs regarding CoNS species[91].

## REFERENCES

[1] Hugonnet, S; Sax, H; Eggimann P; Chevrolet, JC; Pittet, D. Nosocomial bloodstream infection and clinical sepsis. *Emerg Infect Dis.*, 2004,10(1), 76-81.

[2] Menezes, EA; Sá KM; Cunha, FA; Ângelo, MRF; Oliveira, IRN, Salviano, MNC. Frequência e percentual de suscetibilidade de bactérias isoladas em pacientes atendidos na unidade de terapia intensiva do Hospital Geral de Fortaleza. *J Bras Patol Med Lab.*,2007,43(3), 149-155.

[3] Diekema, DJ;Beekmann SE; Chapin, KC; Morel, KA; Munson, E; Doern, GV. Epidemiology and outcome of nosocomial and community-onset bloodstream infection. *J Clin Microbiol.*, 2003,41(8), 3655-60.

[4] Wisplinghoff, H; Bischoff, T;Tallent, SM; Seifert, H; Wenzel, RP; Edmond, MB. Nosocomial bloodstream infections in US hospitals: analysis of 24,179 cases from a prospective nationwide surveillance study. *Clin Infec Dis.*, 2004,39(3), 309-14.

[5] Osuchowski, MF; Welch, K; Siddiqui, J;Remick, DG. Circulating cytokine/inhibitor profiles reshape the understanding of the SIRS/CARS continuum in sepsis and predict mortality. *J Immunol.*, 2006,177(3), 1967-74.

[6] Vandepitte, J;Engbaek, K;Piot P;Heuck, CC;Levanon, Y. *Procedimentos laboratoriais em bacteriologia clínica*. São Paulo, SP: Editora Santos, 1997.

[7] Weinstein, MP; Towns ML; Quartey, SM; Mirrett, S; Reimer, LG; Parmigiani, G; Reller, LB. The clinical significance of positive blood cultures in the 1990s: a prospective comprehensive evaluation of the microbiology, epidemiology, and outcome of bacteremia and fungemia in adults. *Clin InfectDis.*,1997, 24(4), 584-602.

[8] Banderó Filho, VC;Reschke, CR;Horner, R. Perfil epidemiológico das infecções hospitalares na unidade de terapia intensiva infantil do hospital de caridade e beneficência de Cachoeira do Sul, RS. *RBAC*, 2006, 38, 267-70.

[9] Murphy, SL. Deaths: final data for 1998. *Natl Vital Stat Rep.*, 2000, 48(11), 1-105.

[10] Angus, DC;Linde-Zwirble, WT;Lidicker J; Clermont, G;Carcillo J;Pinsky, MR. Epidemiology of severe sepsis in the United States: analysis of incidence, outcome, and associated costs of care. *Crit Care Med.*, 2001, 29(7), 1303-10.

[11] ILAS.Instituto Latino Americano para Estudos da Sepse. *Sepse: um problema de saúde pública*. Brasília, DF: SBM.2015.

[12] Silva, E; Pedro, MA;Sogayar, AC;Mohovic, T; Silva, CL;Janiszewski, M; Cal, RG; de Sousa, EF; Abe, TP; de Andrade, J; de Matos, JD; Rezende, E; Assunção, M;Avezum, A; Rocha, PC; de Matos, GF; Bento, AM; Corrêa, AD; Vieira, PC, Knobel, E. Brazilian Sepsis Epidemiological Study (BASES study). *Crit Care.*, 2004, 8(4), 251-60.

[13] Hall, MJ; Williams, SN; De Frances, CJ;Golosinskiy, A.Inpatient care for septicemia or sepsis: A challenge for patients and hospitals. *NCHS Data Brief,.*2011, 62, 1-8.

[14] Lagu, T; Rothberg, MB; Shieh, MS;Pekow, PS, Steingrub, JS;Lindenauer, PK. Hospitalizations, costs, and outcomes of severe sepsis in the United States 2003 to 2007. *Crit Care Med.*, 2012, 40(3), 754-61.

[15] Linden, PK. Clinical implications of nosocomial Gram-positive bacteremia and superimposed antimicrobial resistance. *Am J Med.*, 1998, 104(5A), 24S-33S.

[16] Pfaller, MA; Jones, RN; Doern, GV;Kugler, K. Bacterial pathogens isolated from patients with bloodstream infection: frequencies of occurrence and antimicrobial susceptibility patterns from the SENTRY antimicrobial surveillance program (United States and Canada, 1997). *Antimicrob Agents Chemother.*,1998, 42(7), 1762-70.

[17] Hidron, AI; Edwards, JR; Patel J; Horan, TC; Sievert, DM; Pollock, DA; Fridkin, SK. NHSN. Annual Update: Antimicrobial-Resistant Pathogens Associated with Healthcare-associated infections: Annual Summary of Data Reported to the National Healthcare Safety Network at the Centers for Disease Control and Prevention, 2006-2007. *Infect Control Hosp Epidemiol.*, 2008, 29(11), 996-1011.

[18] Sievert, DM; Ricks, P; Edwards, JR; Schneider, A; Patel J, Srinivasan, A, Kallen, A; Limbago, B; Fridkin, S. Antimicrobial-resistant pathogens associated with healthcare-associated infections: summary of data reported to the National Healthcare Safety Network at the Centers for Disease Control and Prevention, 2009-2010. *Infect. Control Hosp. Epidemiol.*, 2013, 34(1), 1-14.

[19] Marra, AR; Camargo, LF; Pignatari, AC; Sukiennik, T; Behar, PR; Medeiros, EA; Ribeiro, J; Girão, E; Correa, L; Guerra, C; Brites, C; Pereira, CA;Carneiro, I; Reis, M; Souza, MA; Tranchesi, R; Barata, CU; Edmond, MB.Brazilian SCOPE Study Group.Nosocomial bloodstream infections in Brazilian hospitals: analysis of 2,563 cases from a prospective nationwide surveillance study. *J Clin Microbiol.*; 2011; 49(5); 1866-71.

[20] Assis, DB; Madalosso, G; Ferreira, SA; Yassuda, YY. Análise dos dados do Sistema de Vigilância de Infecção Hospitalar do Estado de São Paulo - Ano 2010. Centro de Vigilância Epidemiológica, Secretaria da Saúde do Estado de São Paulo. Available:< http://www.cve.saude. sp.gov.br/htm/ih/pdf/ih11-dados10.pdf>. Accessed February 2016.

[21] Al-Tawfiq, JA; Sufi, I. Infective endocarditis at a hospital in Saudi Arabia: epidemiology; bacterial pathogens and outcome. *Ann Saudi Med.*,2009,29,433-6.

[22] Ge, Y; Liu, XQ;Xu, YC;Xu, S; Yu, MH, Zhang, W; Deng, GH. Blood collection procedures influence contamination rates in blood culture: a prospective study. *Chin Med J (Engl).*, 2011, 124(23), 4002-6.

[23] Cortes, JA; Leal, AL;Montañez, AM;Buitrago, G; Castillo, JS; Guzman, L;GREBO. Frequency of microorganisms isolated in patients with bacteremia in intensive care units in Colombia and their resistance profiles. *Braz J Infect Dis.*, 2013, 17(3), 346-52.

[24] Euzéby, JP. List of Prokaryotic names with Standing in Nomenclature. Available: <http://www.bacterio.net/s/staphylococcus.html>. Accessed February 2016.

[25] Ferreira, AM;Bonesso, MF; Mondelli, AL; Cunha, MLRS. Identification of *Staphylococcus saprophyticus* isolated from patients with urinary tract infection using a simple set of biochemical tests correlating with 16S-23S interspace region molecular weight patterns. *J Microbiol Methods.*, 2012, 91(3), 406-411.

[26] Mack, D;Sabottke, A;Dobinsky, S; Rohde, H;Horstkotte, MA;Knobloch, KM. Differential expression of methicillin resistance by different biofilm-negative *S. epidermidis* Transposon mutant classes. *Antimicrob. AgentsChemother.*, 2002, 46(1), 178-183.

[27] Morales, M;Méndez-Alvarez, S; Martín-López, JV;Marrero, C;Freytes, CO. Biofilm: the microbial "bunker" for intravascular cateter-related infection. *Support Care Cancer.*, 2004, 12(10), 701-7.

[28] Kloos, WE; Bannerman, TL. Update on clinical Significance of coagulase-negative staphylococci. *Clin Microbiol Rev.*, 1994, 7(1), 117-40.
[29] Heikens, E; Fleer, A;Paauw, A;Florijn, A;Fluit, AC. Comparison of genotypic and phenotypic methods for species level identification of clinical isolates of coagulase-negative staphylococci. *J Clin Microbiol.*, 2005, 43(5), 2286-90.
[30] Archer, GL;Climo, MW. *Staphylococcus epidermidis* and other coagulase negative staphylococci. In: Mandel, GL; Bennett, JE; Dolin, R editors. Principles and practice of infectious diseases. Philadelphia. Elsevier Churchill Livingston, 2005, 2352-62.
[31] Kloos, WE; Bannerman, TL. *Staphylococcus* and *Micrococcus*. In: Murray, PR; Baron, EJ;Pfalle,r MA;Tenove,r FC;Yolken, RH editors. Manual of Clinical Microbiology. Washington: American Society Microbiology, 1999, 264-82.
[32] Rowlinson, MC; LeBourgeois, P; Ward, K; Song, Y;Finegold, SM; Bruckner, DA. Isolation of a Strictly Anaerobic Strain of *Staphylococcus epidermidis*. *J Clin Microbiol.*, 2006, 44(3), 857-60.
[33] Spanu, T;Sanguinetti, M;Ciccaglione, D;D'Inzeo, T; Romano, L; Leone, F;Fadda, G. Use of the VITEK 2 system for rapid identification of clinical isolates of staphylococci from bloodstream infections. *J. Clin. Microbiol.*, 2003, 41(9), 4259-4263.
[34] Rogers, KL; Fey, PD; Rupp, ME. Coagulase-negative staphylococcal infections. *Infect. Dis. Clin. North Am.*,2009, 23(1), 73-98.
[35] Fernandes, AP; Silva, CJ; Costa, C;Schreiber, AZ; Mello, FA; Teixeira-Loyola, ABA. Incidência bacteriana em hemoculturas no hospital das clínicas Samuel Libânio de Pouso Alegre MG. *RevistaEletrônicaAcervo Saúde*, 2011, 2, 122-33.
[36] Gill, SR;Fouts, DE; Archer, GL;Mongodim, EF;Deboy, RT; Ravel, J. Insights on evolution of virulence and resistance from the complete genome analysis of an early methicillin-resistance *Staphylococcus aureus* strain and a biofilm-producing methicillin-resistance *Staphylococcus epidermidis* strain. *J Bacteriol.*, 2005, 187(7), 2426-38.
[37] Schuenck, RP; Pereira, EM;Iorio, NL; Dos Santos, KR. Multiplex PCR assay to identify methicillin-resistant *Staphylococcus haemolyticus*.*FEMS Immunol Med Microbiol.*,2008, 52(3), 431-435.

[38] Ing, MB;Baddour, LM;Baye,r AS. Bacteremia and infective endocarditis: pathogenesis, diagnosis, and complications. In: Crossley, KB; Archer, GL editors. The staphylococci in human disease. New York: Churchill Livingstone, 1997, 331-54.
[39] Takeuchi, F; Watanabe, S; Baba, T;Yuzawa, H; Ito, T; Morimoto, Y; Kuroda, M; Cui, L; Takahashi, M;Ankai, A;Bab,a S; Fukui, S; Lee, JC;Hiramatsu, K. Whole-Genome Sequencing of *Staphylococcus haemolyticus* Uncovers the Extreme Plasticity of Its Genome and the Evolution of Human-Colonizing Staphylococcal Species. *J. Bacteriol.*, 187(21), 2005, 7292-308.
[40] Falcone, M;Giannella, M;Raponi, G; Mancini, C;Venditti,M. Teicoplanin use and emergence of *Staphylococcus haemolyticus*: is there a link? *Clin Microbiol Infect.*, 2006, 12(1), 96-7.
[41] Keim, LS; Torres-Filho, SR; Silva, PV; Teixeira, LA. Prevalence, aetiology and antibiotic resistance profiles of coagulase-negative staphylococci isolated in a teaching hospital. *Braz J Microbiol.*, 2011, 42(1), 248-55.
[42] Kessler, RB; Kimbrough, RC; Jones SR. Infective endocarditis caused by *S. hominis* after vasectomy. *Clin Infect Dis.*, 1998, 27(1), 216-217.
[43] Chaves, F;García-Álvarez, M;Sanz, F; Alba, C; Otero, JR. Nosocomial spread of a *Staphylococcus hominis* subsp. novobiosepticus strain causing sepsis in a neonatal intensive care unit. *J Clin Microbiol.*, 2005, 43(9)4877-4879.
[44] Götz F. The genera *Staphylococcus* and *Micrococcus*. In: Dworkin, M;Falkow, S;Rosenberig, E;Schleiferr, K-H, Stackebrands, editors. The Prokaryotes. A Handbook on the biology of bacteria: Firmicutes, Cyanobacteria.Germany: Springer, 2006, 5-75.
[45] Sorlozano, A; Gutierrez, J; Martinez, T;Yuste, ME; Perez-Lopez, JA;Vindel, A; Guillen, J;Boquete, T. Detection of new mutations conferring resistance to linezolid in glycopeptideintermediate susceptibility *Staphylococcus hominis* subspecies hominis circulating in an intensive care unit. *Eur J Clin Microbiol Infect Dis.*, 2010, 29(1), 73-80.
[46] Bouchami, O; Ben,Hassen, A; de Lencastre, H;Miragaia, M. Molecular epidemiology of methicillin-resistant *Staphylococcus hominis* (MRSHo): low clonality and reservoirs of SCCmec structural elements. *PLoSOne.*, 2011, 6(7), e21940.

[47] Kloos, WE;Schleifer, KH. Isolation and characterization of staphylococci from human skin. II. Description of four new species: *Staphylococcus warneri*;*Staphylococcus capitis*;*Staphylococcus hominis*; and *Staphylococcus simulans*.*Int J SystBacteriol.*, 1975, 25, 62-79.
[48] Nalmas, S;Bishburg, E;Meurillio, J;Khoobiar, S, Cohen, M. *Staphylococcus capitis* prosthetic valve endocarditis: report of two rare cases and review of literature. *Heart Lung.*, 2008, 37(5), 380-384.
[49] Oren, I;Merzbach, D. Clinical and epidemiological significance of species identification of coagulase-negative staphylococci in a microbiological laboratory. *Isr. J. Med. Sci.*, 1990, 26(3), 125-128.
[50] Tristan, A; Lina, G; Etienne, J;Vandenesch, F. Biology and pathogenicity of staphylococci other than *Staphylococcus aureus* and *Staphylococcus epidermidis*. In: Fischetti, VA;Novick, RP;Ferretti, JJ;Portnoy, DA; Rood. JI editors. Gram- positive pathogens. Washington, DC: ASM Press, 2000.
[51] Washington, JA. An international multicenter study of blood culture practices. The International Collaborative Blood Culture Study Group. *Eur J Clin Microbiol Infect Dis.*, 1992, 11(12), 1115-28.
[52] Veronesi, R. 1999. Sepse. In: Tratado de Infectologia. São Paulo: Atheneu.
[53] Gonzalez, BE; Mercado, CK; Johnson, L; Brodsky, NL; Bhandari, V.Early markers of late-onset sepsis in premature neonates: clinical, hematological and cytokine profile.*J Perinat Med.*, 2003, 31(1), 60-8.
[54] Melo, WA; Silva, JO. Sepse - The importance of clinical laboratory the diagnosis. *Rev Saúde Publ.*, 2009, 1, 34-50.
[55] Doern, GV;Vautour, R;Gaudet, M; Levy, B. Clinical impact of rapid in vitro susceptibility testing and bacterial identification. *J Clin Microbiol.*, 1994, 32(7), 1757-62.
[56] Harbarth, S;Garbino, J;Pugin, J;Romand, JA; Lew, D; Pittet, D. Inappropriate initial antimicrobial therapy and its effect on survival in a clinical trial of immunomodulation therapy for severe sepsis. *Am J Med.*, 2003, 115(7), 529-35.
[57] Diament, D; Salomão, R;Rigatto, O; Gomes, B; Silva, E; Carvalho, NB; Machado, FR. Guidelines for the treatment of severe sepsis and septic shock - management of the infectious agent - diagnosis. *Rev Bras TerIntensiva.*,2011,23(2)134-44.

[58] Rivers, E; Nguyen, B;Havstad, S;Ressler, J;Muzzin, A;Knoblich, B; Peterson, E;Tomlanovich, M. Early goal-directed therapy in the treatment of severe sepsis and septic shock. *N Engl J Med.*, 2001, 345(19), 1368-77.

[59] Dellinger, RP;Carlet, JM;Masur, H;Gerlach, H;Calandra, T; Cohen, J;Gea-Banacloche, J;Keh, D; Marshall, JC; Parker, MM; Ramsay, G; Zimmerman, JL; Vincent, JL; Levy, MM. Surviving sepsis campaign guidelines for management of severe sepsis and septic shock. *Crit Care Med.*, 2004, 32(3), 858-73. Review. Erratum in: *Crit Care Med.*, 2004, 32(10), 2169-70. Dosage error in article text.

[60] Gao, F; Melody, T; Daniels, DF; Giles, S; Fox, S. The impact of compliance with 6-hour and 24-hour sepsis bundles on hospital mortality in patients with severe sepsis: a prospective observational study. *Crit Care.*, 2005, 9(6), 764-70.

[61] Kumar, A; Roberts, D; Wood, KE; Light, B;Parrillo, JE; Sharma, S;Suppes, R; Feinstein, D;Zanotti, S;Taiberg, L;Gurka, D; Kumar, A;Cheang, M. Duration of hypotension before initiation of effective antimicrobial therapy is the critical determinant of survival in human septic shock. *Crit Care Med.*, 2006, 34(6), 1589-96.

[62] Höffken, G; Niederman, MS. Nosocomial pneumonia: the importance of a de-escalating strategy for antibiotic treatment of pneumonia in the ICU. *Chest.*,2002, 122(6), 2183-96.

[63] Turnidge, JohnImpact of antibiotic resistance on the treatment of sepsis. *Scand J Infect Dis.*, 2003, 35(9), 677-82.

[64] Niederman, MS. The importance of de-escalating antimicrobial therapy in patients with ventilator-associated pneumonia. *SeminRespir Crit Care Med.*, 2006, 27(1), 45-50.

[65] Barenfanger, J; Drake, C;Kacich, G. Clinical and financial benefits of rapid bacterial identification and antimicrobial susceptibility testing. *J Clin Microbiol.*, 1999, 37(5), 1415-8.

[66] Seifert, H. The clinical importance of microbiological findings in the diagnosis and management of bloodstream infections. *Clin Infect Dis.*, 2009, 15(48) Suppl 4, S238-45.

[67] Woo, PC; Ng, KH; Lau, SK; Yip, KT; Fung, AM; Leung, KW; Tam, DM;Que, TL; Yuen, KY. Usefulness of the microseq 500 16S ribossomaldna-based bacterial identification system for identification of clinically significant bacterial isolates with ambiguous biochemical profiles. *J Clin Microbiol.*, 2003, 41(5), 1996-2001.

[68] Woo, PC; Lau, SK;Teng, JL;Tse, H, Yuen, KY. Then and now: use of 16S rDNA gene sequencing for bacterial identification and discovery of novel bacteria in clinical microbiology laboratories. *Clin Microbiol Infect.*, 2008, 14(10), 908-34.

[69] Pereira, EM;Schuenck, RP;Malvar, KL;Lorio, NLP; Matos, PDM;Olendzki, NA;Oelemann, WMR; Santos, KRN. *Staphylococcus aureus, Staphylococcus epidermidis* and *Staphylococcus haemolyticus*: Methicilin-resistant isolates are detected directly in blood culture by multiplex PCR. *Microbiol Research.*, 2010, 165(3), 243-9.

[70] Reller, L; Murray, P;Maclowery, J. *Blood culture II.* Washington: ASM Press, 1982.

[71] Sader, HS; Jones, RN; Gales, AC; Silva, JB; Pignatari, AC. SENTRY Participants Group (Latin America). SENTRY antimicrobial surveillance program report: Latin America and Brazilian results for 1997 through 2001. *Bras J Infect Dis.*, 2004, 8(1), 25-79.

[72] Tornsberry C. Automated procedures for antimicrobial susceptibility test. In:Manual of clinical microbiology. Washington: ASM Press, 1985.

[73] Stager, CE; Davis, JR. Automated systems for identification of microorganisms. *Clin Microbiol Rev.*, 1992, 5(3), 302-2.

[74] Funke, G; Monnet, D; deBernardis, C; vonGraevenitz, A;Freney, J. Evaluation of the VITEK 2 system for rapid identification of medically relevant gram-negative rods. *J Clin Microbiol.*, 1998, 36(7), 1948-52.

[75] Wallet, F;Loïez, C;Renaux, E; Lemaitre, N;Courcol RJ. Performances of VITEK 2 colorimetric cards for identification of Gram-positive and Gram-negative bacteria. *J Clin Microbiol.*2005, 43(9), 4402-6.

[76] Tomfohrde KM. Review criteria for assessment of antimicrobial susceptibility devices: what do they mean? *Clin Microbiol Newsl.*, 1991, 8:1-8.

[77] Ferraro, MJ; Jorgensen, JH. Instrument-based antibacterial susceptibility testing. In Murray, PR; Baron, EJ; Pfaller, MA; Tenover, LC;Yolken, LH. Manual of clinical microbiology. Washington: American Society for Microbiology, 1995, 1375-84.

[78] Kim, M;Heo, SR; Choi, SH; Kwon, H; Park, JS;Seong, MW; Lee, DH; Park, KU; Song, J; Kim, EC. Comparison of the MicroScan, VITEK 2 and Crystal GP with 16S rRNA sequencing and MicroSeq 500 v2.0 analysis for coagulase-negative Staphylococci. *BMC Microbiol.*, 2008, 23 (8), 233-9.

[79] Delmas, J;Chacornac, JP; Robin, F;Giammarinaro, P; Talon, R; Bonnet, R. Evaluation of the Vitek 2 system with a variety of *Staphylococcus* species. *J Clin Microbiol.*, 2008, 46(1), 311-3.

[80] Paim, TG; Cantarelli, VV; d'Azevedo, PA. Performance of the Vitek 2 system software version 5.03 in the bacterial identification and antimicrobial susceptibility test: evaluation study of clinical and reference strains of Gram-positive cocci. *Rev Soc Bras Med Trop.*, 2014, 47(3), 377-81.

[81] Ligozzi, M; Bernini, C;Bonora, MG;de Fatima, M;Zuliani, J; Fontana, R. Evaluation of the VITEK 2 system for identification and antimicrobial susceptibility testing of medically relevant Gram-positive cocci. *J Clin Microbiol.*, 2002, 40(5), 1681-6.

[82] Available < http://www.biomerieux.com.br>. [Accessed February 2016].

[83] Maier, T; Schwarz, G;Kostrzewa, M. Rapid identification of bacteria from blood cultures using MALDI-TOF MS. Paper presented at the 48th Interscience Conferenceon Antimicrobial Agents and Chemotherapy. Washington: American Society for Microbiology. Abstract D-302, 2008.

[84] Stevenson, LG; Drake, SK; Murray PR. Rapid identification of bacteria in positive blood culture broths by matrix-assisted laser desorption ionization-time of flight mass spectrometry.*J Clin Microbiol.*, 2010, 48(2), 444-7

[85] Szabados, F;Michels, M;Kaase, M;Gatermann, S. The sensitivity of direct identification from positive BacT/ALERT™ (bioMérieux) blood culture bottles by matrix-assisted laser desorption ionization time-of-flight mass spectrometry is low. *Clin Microbiol Infect.*, 2001,17(2), 192-5.

[86] Deng J; Fu L; Wang R; Yu N; Ding X; Jiang L; Fang Y; Jiang C; Lin L; Wang Y;Che X. Comparison of MALDI-TOF MS; gene sequencing and the Vitek 2 for identification of seventy-three clinical isolates of enteropathogens. *J Thorac Dis.*, 2014, 6(5), 539-44.

[87] Winn Jr, WC; Allen, SD;Janda, WM; Koneman, EW;Procop, GW;Schreckenberger, PC; Woods, GL. In:*Koneman. Diagnóstico microbiológico: texto e atlas colorido.* Rio de Janeiro:Guanabara-Koogan, 2010.

[88] Millar, B; Moore, J; Mallon, P;Xu, J; Crowe M;Macclurg, R;Raoult, D; Earle J; Hone, R;Murphy, P. Molecular diagnosis of infective endocarditis - a new Duke´s criterion. *Scand J Infect Dis.*, 2001, 33(9), 673-680.

[89] Kolbert C P;Persing DH. Ribosomal DNA sequencing as a tool for identification of bacterial pathogens. *Curr Opin Microbiol.*, 1999, 2(3), 299-305.

[90] Patel, JB. 16S rRNA gene sequencing for bacterial pathogen identification in the clinical laboratory. *Mol Diagn.*, 2001, 6(4), 313-21.

[91] Hogg, GM.; McKenna, JP; Ong, G. Rapid detection of methicillin-susceptible and methicillin-resistant *Staphylococcus aureus* directly from positive BacT/Alert blood culture bottles using real-time polymerase chain reaction: evaluation and comparison of 4 DNA extraction methods. *Diagn Microbiol Infect Dis.*, 2008, 61(4), 446-52.

In: *Staphylococcus aureus*
Editor: M. L. R. S. Cunha

ISBN: 978-1-63485-959-2
© 2017 Nova Science Publishers, Inc.

*Chapter 6*

# STAPHYLOCOCCUS AUREUS INFECTIONS IN NEWBORNS

*Danilo Flávio Moraes Riboli, Thaís Alves Barbosa and Maria de Lourdes Ribeiro de Souza da Cunha*[*]

Department of Microbiology and Immunology, Botucatu Institute of Biosciences, UNESP - Univ Estadual Paulista, Botucatu, São Paulo State, Brazil

## ABSTRACT

The prevention and control of bacterial infections in newborns represents a challenge for health professionals. Outbreaks of infection in premature newborns (NBs), after colonization, have been widely reported to cause large numbers of deaths. It is known that in neonates, bacterial colonization begins shortly after birth, characterized by the presence of the microorganism in the host without clinical manifestations or immune responses. The primary risk factors for infection in NBs include colonization, prematurity, low birth weight, immaturity of the immune system, prolonged hospital stays, the use of antimicrobials and invasive procedures and/or surgery. Among the pathogens most commonly associated with colonization and infection in Neonatal Intensive Care Units (NICU) are the species of the *Staphylococcus* genus, among which *Staphylococcus aureus* is considered the most important pathogen of the genus, able to cause numerous infectious processes with multiple clinical

---

[*] Corresponding author: cunhamlr@ibb.unesp.br

symptomatologies, from localized diseases to systemic frameworks. The methicillin-resistant *Staphylococcus aureus* (MRSA) is included as an integral part of this group, one of the main pathogens in nosocomial infections, with prevalence of 1.5% in neonates in NICUs and 3% in children in Pediatric Intensive Care Units. In catheter related bloodstream infections, the Centers of Disease Control data report the coagulase-negative staphylococci as the most common pathogens, followed by *S. aureus*, *Enterococcus* and *Candida* species. Neonatal sepsis is classified according to the onset of the disease. It is called early onset when it occurs in the first week of life, and late onset when it occurs between the first week and the end of the neonatal period and can be defined clinically, diagnosed through a combination of clinical signs (such as thermal instability, bradycardia, apnea, hypoactivity/lethargy, food intolerance), and/or microbiologically confirmed through laboratory tests and detection of bacteria in the blood culture. Together with the sepsis syndrome, meningitis can occur both early and late and the clinical presentation may be indistinguishable from neonatal sepsis. Due to the clinical importance, increased morbidity and mortality, this chapter aims at discussing the epidemiological role of *S. aureus* in infections in NBs, through colonization, pathogenicity, diagnosis and treatment.

# INTRODUCTION

According to World Health Organization estimates, there are about 5 million deaths of newborns per year, 98% of them in developing countries [1]. In these countries, neonatal mortality (deaths in the first 28 days of life per 1000 live births) from all causes is about 34; in contrast, neonatal mortality in developed countries is about 5, many of these deaths occur in the first week of life, the majority on the first day [2].

The most common causes of death in the neonatal period are infections, including sepsis, meningitis, respiratory infections, diarrhea and tetanus (32%), followed by birth asphyxia and injuries (29%) and prematurity (24%) [2].

Nosocomial infections are manifested intensely and frequently in newborns (NBs) when compared to children or adults. In addition to the different needs of this age group, which make them more sensitive to the acquisition of infection, numerous invasive procedures, the use of broad-spectrum antimicrobials and the extension of the period of stay in the Neonatal Intensive Care Unit (NICU) are factors that may lead to hospital-acquired neonatal infections [3].

The prevention and control of bacterial infections in newborns symbolize a challenge for all health professionals. Outbreaks of infection after colonization have been widely reported to cause a substantial proportion of neonatal deaths [1]. Colonized children can serve as an endogenous reservoir for cross-transmission of microorganisms and are often identified as the source of outbreaks in the NICU and Pediatric Intensive Care Unit (PICU) [4], however, their family and the professional team can play an important role in the transmission chain [5].

## COLONIZATION AND INFECTION

The process of colonization is characterized by the presence of the microorganism in the host in the absence of clinical manifestations and immune response at the moment of bacterial isolation [6].

The developing fetus is protected from maternal microbiota. The normal colonization process in NBs begins subsequent to rupture of the amniotic membrane, continuing through contact with the mother and the environment until the microbiota of the baby is established. Several factors may influence the colonization process in the neonate, among them the maternal microbiota, feeding of the newborn, people who establish direct contact with the child and the environment in which it is born and remains, comprising objects and microbiota of other babies who occupy the same space [7].

Often NBs who maintain contact with the mother and are breastfed are subsequently colonized at birth through the skin and mucosal surfaces, such as the nasopharynx, oropharynx, conjunctiva, external genitalia and umbilical cord [6]. The presence of some virulent microbiota protect the child's colonization from potentially pathogenic micro-organisms, as bacteria of the microbiota proliferate in various sites, competing with pathogenic organisms, with lower proportions of progression to disease [3].

Premature neonates who remain in intensive care are susceptible to colonization by microorganisms as a result of treatment with antibiotics, parenteral nutrition and staying in incubators; such facts may delay or hinder the normal intestinal colonization process, serving as a potential source for invasive infection [8].

Infection characterized by the invasion of microorganisms that multiply and cause damage usually manifests itself by the direct expansion of colonization sites or invasion of the bloodstream, resulting in the spread of the infectious process, depending on the virulence of the pathogen, the inoculum and the interaction between the pathogen and host [3].

The primary risk factors for infection in newborns can be divided into intrinsic and extrinsic. Intrinsic factors include characteristics such as gender, birth weight, gestational age, degree of immune development and disease severity [9]. Extrinsic factors include duration of hospitalization, use of invasive procedures (tracheal tubes, arterial and venous catheters, gastric or duodenal probes, ventricular-peritoneal shunts, chest drains, etc.), peculiarities of exposure to the hospital environment and the multidisciplinary team, and the unit's method of using antimicrobials [10, 11]. As the population of NICU patients increases, due to viability limits being pushed for increasingly lower gestational age and the rapid advance in technology, enabling the survival of babies, there is a possibility that many infants are at risk of being colonized and infected with MRSA [12].

Predisposition to acquire an infectious process stems from a combination of several risk factors as a consequence of the immaturity of the immune system and the disruption of normal defense barriers. Thus newborns submitted to the use of endotracheal cannulas and mechanical ventilators which interfere with the mechanisms of local pulmonary defense, the use of catheters that favor the entry of skin microflora bacteria into the bloodstream, mechanisms which lead to reduced gastric acidity with the use of H2 blockers, and enteral hyperalimentation may cause the placement of pathogenic organisms and the use of prolonged and routine antimicrobials, whose selective pressure enables colonization by resistant microorganisms. Infections caused by multidrug-resistant microorganisms are a severe challenge in newborns admitted to the NICU, with an established relationship with rising mortality rates, morbidity, increased hospital stay and the risk of neurological sequel in the long-term [13]. Thus, the extension of the period in the NICU favors colonization by potentially pathogenic microorganisms, favoring the development of healthcare associated infections (HAIs) [3].

The development of sepsis and meningitis in newborns has been linked to various risk factors in the mother and the newborn. Perinatal and intrauterine infections and maternal urinary tract infections have repeatedly been associated with neonatal meningitis [14-16]. Other reported risk factors are prematurity, prolonged rupture of membranes, and low birth weight [15-17]. Many of these factors are associated with the interference of the physical barriers that protect the newborn during the perinatal period from infections caused by maternal microbiota. The route of infection may be hematogenous (placenta) or by direct inoculation of pathogens (aspiration/inhalation). With the development of bacteremia, microorganisms can gain access to cerebrospinal fluid [17].

Meningitis can occur as part of a septic syndrome both early and late onset or as a focal infection. In some studies, the incidence of bacterial meningitis in neonates ranges from 0.25 to 1 per 1,000 live births [14, 16, 18]. However, in a review study, the incidence of neonatal meningitis ranged from 0.8 to 6.1 per 1,000 live births [19]. Historically, in neonates with bacterial sepsis and positive blood cultures, more than 25% will also have meningitis confirmed by culture [20].

The clinical presentation of neonatal meningitis is often sudden and indistinguishable from neonatal sepsis without meningitis. The most commonly reported symptoms are fever, irritability and poor feeding [21, 22].

The microorganisms most frequently found in meningitis in newborns include *S. aureus*, *Streptococcus viridans* and Coagulase-negative Staphylococci (CoNS). These Gram-positive microorganisms are commonly found in preterm newborns or related to medical devices [23]. However; the etiology of neonatal meningitis in developing countries is different from that of developed countries. In the majority of developed countries, the predominant pathogens isolated from the cerebrospinal fluid in newborns are Group B *Streptococcus* (GBS), *E. coli*, *Listeria monocytogenes*, other Gram-negative enterobacteria and *Streptococcus pneumonie* [24-26].

Infections in the neonatal period are often divided into early (first 5-7 days, implying vertical transmission) in which GBS, *E. coli* and *Listeria monocytogenes* bacteria are often isolated and late (after the first week of life), implying community or nosocomially acquired infection, which include *Staphylococcus* spp. and Gram negative bacilli [27].

The definition of bloodstream infection includes both clinical sepsis and laboratory confirmed infection. Clinical sepsis is defined as the worsening of the condition of the NB caused by microorganisms or toxins in the blood with clinical evidence of infection; a positive blood culture for known pathogens is not necessary [9].

It is confirmed microbiologically by positive blood and/or cerebrospinal fluid cultures and can be classified according to the disease onset: early or late. The difference between the two is of clinical relevance, early onset infection occurs mainly through bacteria acquired before and during delivery and is conventionally considered as acquired from the mother with disease-causing microorganisms commonly found in the maternal genital tract, and late onset infection through bacteria after delivery with a nosocomial or community source [28].

In the case of laboratory confirmed bloodstream infection, two positive blood cultures are required for skin contaminants unrelated to infections in other locations. The infection is classified as secondary when the microorganism is found in another location, with the exception of those related to a catheter, which are classified as primary [28].

In a study conducted in Portugal over 75 years in an NICU, the average time of onset of sepsis was 19 days. Total mortality in the study population was 22% and mortality in sepsis cases was approximately 12% in the total study period for all summed microorganisms. The mortality rate related to sepsis fell steadily over the 75 years from 87% in 1928 to 3% in 2003. Specifically, the mortality rate for *S. aureus* was 13% and CoNS 5% [29].

An interesting fact related to the cause of sepsis in that study was the continued growth of commensal species, reaching 44% of the microorganisms responsible for cases of sepsis. Episodes caused by CoNS increased from 8 to 29% and *S. aureus* from 3 to 8% [29]. The prevalence of infections by CoNS, especially in late cases of sepsis have already been reported [30, 31]. Prematurity, prolonged intravascular access and mechanical ventilation, and the use of parenteral nutrition and its duration are among the risk factors associated with CoNS infections in NICUs [30, 32].

The most implicated pathogens in neonatal sepsis in developing countries may differ from those found in developed countries. In general, the most common Gram negative microorganisms are *Klebsiella*, *E. coli*, *Pseudomonas* and *Salmonella* [33-35]. Of the Gram-positive microorganisms, *S. aureus* [35-37], CoNS [38], *Streptococcus pneumoniae* and *Streptococcus pyogenes* [39, 40] are the most commonly isolated.

Of the pathogens most commonly associated with infections in NICUs are the species of the *Staphylococcus* genus, among which *Staphylococcus aureus* is considered the most important pathogen of the genus, being a member of the normal microbiota of the skin of humans and other animals [41]. *S. aureus* is considered one of the prevalent virulent agents, able to cause many infectious processes that manifest themselves with different clinical symptomatology, encompassing from localized pathologies to those with a systemic framework [42, 43]. Morphologically, *Staphylococcus* spp. are presented as Gram-positive cocci assembled into structures resembling grape clusters. Within the genus, about 15 of the 52 known species are capable of causing an infectious process in humans. For differentiation from the other members of the genus, *Staphylococcus aureus* can be identified through coagulase production [44].

*Staphylococcus* spp. presents high resistance worldwide [45]. The emergence of methicillin-resistant strains represents a clinically serious problem as the antimicrobial used for infection control has become ineffective. This problem has caused many researchers to elucidate possible mechanisms of resistance to correctly treat the infections, preventing the patient from being treated unnecessarily, leading to selection of resistant strains, since these microorganisms can be diagnosed wrongly, being present as contaminants of samples and materials [46].

Methicillin resistance can be detected using the genotypic technique of polymerase chain reaction (PCR), known as the gold standard for detection of the *mecA* gene. Such resistance is mediated through production of a supplementary penicillin binding protein (PBP) (PBP 2' or PBP 2a), which presents low affinity with semi-synthetic penicillins, the *mec*A gene being the genetic determinant of this protein of chromosomal nature. The *mec*A gene is identified in all *Staphylococcus* species and therefore is a useful molecular marker for resistance to methicillin [47, 48]. The *mec*A gene is located in a mobile genetic element known as the Staphyloccocal Cassette Chromosome *mec* (SCC*mec*) [49]. The SCC*mec* element contains the *mec* gene complex (the *mecA* gene and regulators) and the *ccr* gene complex that encodes site-specific recombinase responsible for the mobility of SCC*mec* [50]. These are classified into types I, II, III, IV, V and VI according to the *mec* and *ccr* gene complexes. Types I, II, III and VI are located distributed in the hospitals and dissemination of these types occurs primarily through selective exposure to antimicrobial pressure related to the time of use. Types IV and V are widely distributed in the strains found in the community and are easily transferred from CoNS to *S. aureus* by presenting small dimensions (21- 28 kbp) in relation to the others [49]. The development and implementation of molecular diagnostic methods, in accordance with infection control policies, and the implementation of decolonization policies with favorable outcomes among pediatric patients are needed as some alternatives in an attempt to control the spread of these microorganisms [51].

As an integral part of this group methicillin-resistant *Staphylococcus aureus* (MRSA) is included, responsible for 19,000 deaths annually [52]. MRSA was first isolated in 1961 by hospital services located in the UK. Since the description of the first case, this microorganism has become increasingly evident as a progressive cause of infections worldwide [52]. Nearly twenty years after the description of the first case, MRSA infection was detected in an NICU. Since then, this pathogen has become evident in infectious processes in premature and severely compromised newborns [53]. These infections are not restricted to skin and soft tissue infections such as mastitis, wound infections and abscesses, but can also be related to symptoms of pneumonia, osteomyelitis, sepsis, lymphadenitis and endocarditis, which cause increased hospitalization time, elevated spending on care and high rates of mortality and morbidity [54].

Studies reveal cases of vertical transmission of MRSA [55]. Research shows that the rate of vaginal MRSA colonization in pregnant women is 2.8%, a fact that suggests the possibility of these women acting as MRSA deposits, transmitting to their offspring through labor [56]. Vertical transmission of MRSA may occur through different methods, such as the birth canal, maternal chorioamnionitis [57], nasal colonization [58] and breastfeeding [58, 59]. Some situations may expose newborns to bacterial colonization by resistant strains, such as the admission of patients who are carriers of these pathogens and prolongation of the hospitalization process. This fact is justified by the possibility of sensitive bacteria developing resistance mechanisms as a result of genetic mutations or through the sharing of resistant genes, as is the case of resistance by induction and selection of resistant bacteria [60].

MRSA has become an extremely important pathogen in community hospitals, long-term care facilities and tertiary hospitals. Generally, these microorganisms can cause a variety of infections in the pediatric population, including bloodstream infections, skin and soft tissue infections, pneumonia, and respiratory tract infections [61-63]. These infections can lead to significant morbidity, including prolonged hospitalization, an increase in the need for more aggressive treatments and the potential for long-term medical problems [12]. Despite advances in neonatal care, as a whole, the rate of death from sepsis can vary from 2 to 50% [20].

Between 30 and 70% of humans are carriers of *S. aureus*, thus, newborns have a high likelihood of exposure during the period immediately after birth [64]. The most common sites of colonization by *S. aureus* include the umbilical cord, skin, nasopharynx, and gastrointestinal tract [64, 65]. For MRSA, the nose and the navel are the most common sites of initial colonization [66].

Moreover, several studies have shown that neonatal colonization by MRSA is a subsequent risk factor for the development of infections by these micro-organisms. Huang et al. [56] found in their study that NBs colonized with MRSA had a significantly higher rate of MRSA infection (26%) when compared with non-colonized NBs (2%).

Traditionally, MRSA has demonstrated a horizontal spread in transmission associated with health care, such as contact with professionals or the hospital environment [4, 67, 68]. Additional factors, such as overcrowding and few professionals in the NICU, have been associated with an increased risk of transmission and colonization, which can lead to MRSA infection outbreaks. Not infrequently, the vertical transmission of MRSA from mothers to their children has been described [55].

Low birth weight has also been associated with increased risk of colonization and/or MRSA infection in several studies [66, 69, 70] as well as prematurity and multiple pregnancies. A variety of procedures and devices used in NICUs are also associated with increasing this risk, including intubation and mechanical ventilation [71], central venous catheterization, parenteral nutrition [66] and surgery [69]. A longer stay in hospital, the kangaroo method of maternal care and the presence of mucus in the eyes of newborns have been shown as independent risk factors for MRSA infection [70].

The prevalence of MRSA colonization and infection rates in NICUs vary widely between institutions due to various factors related to infection control policies, differences in the prevalence of MRSA in the local community, and global differences in MRSA colonization rates. Despite these variations in prevalence, studies have reported values between 0.6% and 8.4% of colonized or infected patients during study periods [12].

One specific study looked at the rate of infection attributed to MRSA after three days of life, in NICUs, participants in a surveillance system of nosocomial infections, for a period of ten years. They found that the incidence of MRSA infections increased by 308%, from 0.7 to 3.1 per 10,000 patient-days, between 1995 and 2004 [61].

In a meta-analysis was found a prevalence of MRSA colonization on admission to the NICU or PICU of 1.9%; among patients in the NICU the prevalence was 1.5%, compared with 3% among patients in the PICU [51]. Children and newborns admitted to an NICU or PICU which carry MRSA were 24.2 times more likely to develop an infection associated with the pathogen during hospitalization compared with non-colonized units. In adult patients, the corresponding figure was 8.3% [72]. The authors also mention the importance of prior colonization in the development of MRSA infections in both populations [51].

Interestingly, the prevalence of MRSA colonization among the babies not born at the study site was 5.8%, compared with only 0.2% among those born in the study hospital, with a statistically significant difference ($P = 0.01$) [51].

The older age of the babies born outside the study hospital [73, 74], which can be translated into more prolonged contact with health professionals during their stay at the previous hospital and their transport to the NICU, could explain this difference. The increase in MRSA colonization on admission could justify the practice of some centers which isolate the population of NBs born elsewhere until their status is known [75, 76].

Maraqa et al. [77] found a relative risk of infection by MRSA for colonized NBs of 37.75 compared to non-colonized NBs, with an average duration of colonization of 20 days. The authors also stated that for each 10-day increase in stay in the NICU, the relative risk of being infected and colonized by MRSA strains increased by 1.32 and 1.29, respectively. The results revealed that the active implementation of surveillance cultures for MRSA identified significantly more affected NBs than clinical cultures alone [77].

In a study conducted in an NICU for 30 months, Conceição et al. [29] analyzed *S. aureus* isolated from NBs (mostly blood cultures and catheters) and surveillance cultures, including health professionals (nasal colonization was 28% among the professionals studied), parents of the children (two were nasal carriers and one of the mothers had the bacteria in the nipple) and the environment of the NICU (a strain was found in plastic folders used to protect clinical files). When analyzed by PFGE, the majority of isolates (70.4%) belonged to three main clones, accounting for 11 of the 16 infected NBs and maintained in the unit during the 30 month study, suggesting that these clones are not only endemic, but also possess high dissemination. The majority of professionals were colonized with clonal types of MSSA endemic in the unit, acting as potentially pathogenic MSSA reservoirs within the NICU. The strain found in the environment was the same as found in the professionals and also the cause of one of the cases of infection that lasted for months. The bacteria found in the nipple of the only mother breastfeeding was the cause of sepsis and abscess in the NB. The NB may have been colonized initially and later developed the infection from an endogenous source, subsequently colonizing the mother, who became a reservoir for the strain [29].

Health professionals and parents of NBs can constitute a bridge between the hospital and the community, and represent possible vehicles for the introduction of isolates related to the community in the NICU. Furthermore, it is known that *S. aureus* can be viable in dry environments, with a 12-day average survival on inanimate surfaces in the ICU [78, 79].

Clinical cultures generally underestimate the prevalence of MRSA in the NICU, while active surveillance cultures are capable of detecting MRSA colonization, and provide information of great help in the control and prevention of MRSA [80]. The surveillance of nosocomial infections is essential to improve the quality of patient care. In an NICU with high rates of endemic MRSA, a set of procedures for infection control proved capable of reducing the colonization rate from over 40% to approximately 10% during the study period [81].

## CONCLUSION

It is important that the medical community continue to monitor and share reports relating to the local prevalence of MRSA strains, the incidence of invasive infections and susceptibility to antibiotics, in an effort to provide cumulative data that can contribute to global awareness and treatment guidelines for this pathogen. Prevention of MRSA transmission in the NICU has shown to be achievable through implementation of appropriate infection control strategies, such as hand hygiene practices; prevention of catheter-related bloodstream infections; sensible use of antimicrobials; skin care, since it is the first barrier of defense against infections; and enteral feeding with human milk as early as possible. To design strategies effective in reducing neonatal sepsis, it is essential to define the sources of infection. Thus, continuous monitoring is essential.

## REFERENCES

[1] Stoll, BJ. The Global Impact of Neonatal Infection. *Clin Perinatol.*, 1997, 24(1), 1–21.
[2] Vergnano, S. Neonatal Sepsis: An International Perspective. *Arch Dis Child Fetal Neonatal.*, 2005, 90(3), F220–f224. doi:10.1136/adc.2002.022863.
[3] Mussi-Pinhata, MM; Nascimento, SD. Neonatal nosocomial infections. *J Pediatr (Rio J).*, 2001, 77(1), S81–96.
[4] Geva, A; Sharon B; Wright, LM; Baldini, JA; Smallcomb, CS; James, EG. Spread of Methicillin-Resistant *Staphylococcus aureus* in a Large Tertiary NICU: Network Analysis. *Pediatrics.*, 2011, 128(5), 1173–80. doi:10.1542/peds.2010-2562.
[5] Giuffrè, M; Celestino, B; Domenico, C; Caterina, M. MRSA Infection in the Neonatal Intensive Care Unit. *Expert Rev Anti Infect Ther.*, 2013, 11(5), 499–509. doi:10.1586/eri.13.28.
[6] Jarvis, WR. The Epidemiology of Colonization. *Infect Control Hosp Epidemiol.*, 1996, 17(1), 47–52.

[7]  Goldmann, DA. The Bacterial Flora of Neonates in Intensive Care-Monitoring and Manipulation. *J Hosp Infect.*, 1988, 11(Suppl A), 340–51.

[8]  Manzoni, P; De Luca, D; Stronati, M; Jacqz-Aigrain, E; Ruffinazzi, G; Luparia, M; Tavella, E; et al. Prevention of Nosocomial Infections in Neonatal Intensive Care Units. *Am J Perinatol.*, 2013, 30(2), 81–88. doi:10.1055/s-0032-1333131.

[9]  Gaynes, RP; Edwards, JR; Jarvis, WR; Culver, DH; Tolson, JS; Martone, WJ. Nosocomial Infections among Neonates in High-Risk Nurseries in the United States. National Nosocomial Infections Surveillance System. *Pediatrics.*, 1996, 98(3 Pt 1), 357–61.

[10] Mullett, MD; Cook, EF; Gallagher, R. Nosocomial Sepsis in the Neonatal Intensive Care Unit. *J Perinatol.*, 1998, 18(2), 112–15.

[11] Asensio, A; Oliver, A; González-Diego, P; Baquero, F; Pérez-Díaz, JC; Ros, P; Cobo, J; Palacios, M; Lasheras, D; Cantón, R. Outbreak of a Multiresistant *Klebsiella pneumoniae* Strain in an Intensive Care Unit: Antibiotic Use as Risk Factor for Colonization and Infection. *Clin Infect Dis.*, 2000, 30(1), 55–60. doi:10.1086/313590.

[12] Nelson, MU; Patrick GG. Methicillin-Resistant *Staphylococcus aureus* in the Neonatal Intensive Care Unit. *Semin Perinatol.*, 2012, 36(6), 424–30. doi:10.1053/j.semperi.2012.06.004.

[13] Sadowska-Krawczenko, I; Jankowska, A; Kurylak, A. Healthcare-Associated Infections in a Neonatal Intensive Care Unit. *Arch Med Sci.*, 2012, 8(5), 854–58. doi:10.5114/aoms.2012.31412.

[14] Bell, AH; Brown, D; Halliday, HL; McClure, G; McReid, M. Meningitis in the Newborn--a 14 Year Review. *Arch Dis Child.*, 1989, 64(6); 873–74. doi:10.1136/adc.64.6.873.

[15] Berman, PH; Banker, BQ. Neonatal Meningitis. A Clinical and Pathological Study of 29 Cases. *Pediatrics.*, 1966, 38(1), 6–24.

[16] Hristeva, L; Booy, R; Bowler, I; Wilkinson, AR. Prospective Surveillance of Neonatal Meningitis. *Arch Dis Child.*,1993, 69(1), 14–18.

[17] de Louvois, J. Acute Bacterial Meningitis in the Newborn. *J Antimicrob Chemother.*, 1994, 34 Suppl A, 61–73.

[18] Franco, SM; Cornelius, VE; Andrews, BF. Long-Term Outcome of Neonatal Meningitis. *Am J Dis Child., (1960)* 1992, 146(5), 567–71.

[19] Thaver, D; Zaidi, AKM. Burden of Neonatal Infections in Developing Countries: A Review of Evidence From Community-Based Studies.

*Pediat Infect Dis J.*, 2009, 28(Supplement), S3–9. doi:10.1097/INF.0b013e3181958755.

[20] Feigin, RD; McCracken, GH; Klein, JO. Diagnosis and Management of Meningitis. *Pediatr Infect Dis J.*, 1992, 11(9), 785–814.

[21] Baumgartner, ET; Augustine, RA; Steele, RW. Bacterial Meningitis in Older Neonates. *Am J Dis Child.*, 1983, 137(11), 1052–54.

[22] Shattuck, KE; Chonmaitree, T. The Changing Spectrum of Neonatal Meningitis over a Fifteen-Year Period. *Clin Pediatr (Phila).*, 1992, 31(3), 130–36.

[23] Gladstone, IM; Ehrenkranz, RA; Edberg, SC; Baltimore, RS. A Ten-Year Review of Neonatal Sepsis and Comparison with the Previous Fifty-Year Experience. *Pediatr Infect Dis J.*, 1990, 9(11), 819–25.

[24] Harvey, D; Holt, DE; Bedford, H. Bacterial Meningitis in the Newborn: A Prospective Study of Mortality and Morbidity. *Semin Perinatol.*, 1999, 23(3), 218–25.

[25] Pong, A; Bradley, JS. Bacterial Meningitis and the Newborn Infant. *Infect Dis Clin North Am.*, 1999, 13(3), 711–33.

[26] Chien, CHY; Chiu, NC; Li, WC; Huang, FY. Characteristics of Neonatal Bacterial Meningitis in a Teaching Hospital in Taiwan from 1984-1997. *J Microbiol Immunol Infect.*, 2000, 33(2), 100–104.

[27] Furyk, JS; Swann, O; Molyneux, E. Systematic Review: Neonatal Meningitis in the Developing World: Neonatal Meningitis in the Developing World. *Trop Med Int Health.*, 2011, 16(6), 672–79. doi:10.1111/j.1365-3156.2011.02750.x.

[28] Nagata, E; Brito, ASJ; Matsuo, T. Nosocomial Infections in a Neonatal Intensive Care Unit: Incidence and Risk Factors. *Am J Infect Control.*, 2002, 30(1), 26–31. doi:10.1067/mic.2002.119823.

[29] Conceição, T; Sousa, MA; Miragaia, M; Paulino, E; Barroso, R; Brito, MJ; Sardinha, T; et al. *Staphylococcus Aureus* Reservoirs and Transmission Routes in a Portuguese Neonatal Intensive Care Unit: A 30-Month Surveillance Study. *Microb Drug Resist.*, 2012, 18(2), 116–24. doi:10.1089/mdr.2011.0182.

[30] Stoll, BJ; Hansen, N; Fanaroff, AA; Wright, LL; Carlo, WA; Ehrenkranz, RA; Lemons, JA; et al. Late-Onset Sepsis in Very Low Birth Weight Neonates: The Experience of the NICHD Neonatal Research Network. *Pediatrics.*, 2002, 110(2), 285–91.

[31] Stoll, BJ; Hansen, N. Infections in VLBW Infants: Studies from the NICHD Neonatal Research Network. *Semin Perinatol.*, 2003, 27(4), 293–301.

[32] Moro, ML; De Toni, A; Stolfi, I; Carrieri, MP; Braga, M; Zunin, C. Risk Factors for Nosocomial Sepsis in Newborn Intensive and Intermediate Care Units. *Eur J Pediatr.*, 1996, 155(4), 315–22.

[33] Moreno, MT; Vargas, S; Poveda, R; Sáez-Llorens, X. Neonatal Sepsis and Meningitis in a Developing Latin American Country. *Pediatr Infect Dis J.*, 1994, 13(6), 516–20.

[34] Tallur, SS; Kasturi, AV; Nadgir, SD; Krishna, BV. Clinico-Bacteriological Study of Neonatal Septicemia in Hubli. *Indian J Pediatr.*, 2000, 67(3), 169–74.

[35] Karthikeyan, G; Premkumar, K. Neonatal Sepsis: *Staphylococcus aureus* as the Predominant Pathogen. *Indian J Pediatr.*, 2001, 68(8), 715–17.

[36] Mulholland, EK; Ogunlesi, OO; Adegbola, RA; Weber, M; Sam, BE; Palmer, A; Manary, MJ; et al. Etiology of Serious Infections in Young Gambian Infants. *Pediatr Infect Dis J.*, 1999, 18(10), S35–41.

[37] Bhutta, ZA; Yusuf, K. Early-Onset Neonatal Sepsis in Pakistan: A Case Control Study of Risk Factors in a Birth Cohort. *Am J Perinatol.*, 1997, 14(9), 577–81. doi:10.1055/s-2007-994338.

[38] Malik, AS; Pennie, RA. Early Onset Neonatal Septicaemia in a Level II Nursery. *Med J Malaysia.*, 1994, 49(1), 17–23.

[39] Muhe, L; Tilahun, M; Lulseged, S; Kebede, S; Enaro, D; Ringertz, S; Kronvall, G; Gove, S; Mulholland, EK. Etiology of Pneumonia, Sepsis and Meningitis in Infants Younger than Three Months of Age in Ethiopia. *Pediatr Infect Dis J.*, 1999, 18(10), S56–61.

[40] Gatchalian, SR; Quiambao, BP; Morelos, AM; Abraham, L; Gepanayao, CP; Sombrero, LT; Paladin, JF; Soriano, VC; Obach, M; Sunico, ES. Bacterial and Viral Etiology of Serious Infections in Very Young Filipino Infants. *Pediatr Infect Dis J.*, 1999, 18(10), S50–55.

[41] Murray, PR; Rosenthal, KS; Pfaller, MA. *Medical Microbiology.* 6th ed. Philadelphia: Mosby/Elsevier. 2009.

[42] Smith, TC; Forshey, BM; Hanson, BM; Wardyn, SE; Moritz, ED. Molecular and Epidemiologic Predictors of *Staphylococcus aureus* Colonization Site in a Population with Limited Nosocomial Exposure. *Am J Infect Control.*, 2012, 40(10), 992–96. doi:10.1016/j.ajic.2011.11.017.

[43] Edwards, AM; Massey, RC; Clarke, SR. Molecular Mechanisms of *Staphylococcus aureus* Nasopharyngeal Colonization. *Mol Oral Microbiol.*, 2012, 27(1), 1–10. doi:10.1111/j.2041-1014.2011.00628.x.

[44] Euzéby, JP. List of Prokaryotic Names with Standing in Nomenclature – Genus *Staphylococcus*. January 28. http://www.bacterio.cict.fr/s/staphylococcus.html. 2016.

[45] Robinson, DA; Enright, MC. Evolutionary Models of the Emergence of Methicillin-Resistant *Staphylococcus aureus*. *Antimicrob Agents Chemother.*, 2003, 47(12), 3926–34.

[46] Alcaráz, LE; Satorres, SE; Lucero, RM; Centorbi, ONP. Species Identification, Slime Production and Oxacillin Susceptibility in Coagulase-Negative Staphylococci Isolated from Nosocomial Specimens. *Braz J Microbiol.*, 2003, 34(1), 45–51. doi:10.1590/S1517-83822003000100010.

[47] Chambers, HF; Hartman, BJ; Tomasz, A. Increased Amounts of a Novel Penicillin-Binding Protein in a Strain of Methicillin-Resistant *Staphylococcus aureus* Exposed to Nafcillin. *J Clin Invest.*, 1985, 76(1), 325–31. doi:10.1172/JCI111965.

[48] Archer, GL; Niemeyer, DM. Origin and Evolution of DNA Associated with Resistance to Methicillin in Staphylococci. *Trends Microbiol.*, 1994, 2(10), 343–47.

[49] Moussallem, BC; Kury, CMH; Medina-Acosta, E. Detecção Dos Genes *mec*A E *fem*A, Marcadores Moleculares de Resistência a Meticilina, Em *Staphylococcus spp*. Isolados de Pacientes Admitidos Em Uma Unidade Neonatal de Tratamento Intensivo. *Revista Científica Da FMC.*, 2007, 2(2), 2–9.

[50] Katayama, Y; Ito, T; Hiramatsu, K. A New Class of Genetic Element, Staphylococcus Cassette Chromosome Mec, Encodes Methicillin Resistance in *Staphylococcus aureus*. *Antimicrob Agents Chemother.*, 2000, 44(6), 1549–55.

[51] Zervou, FN; Zacharioudakis, IM; Ziakas, PD; Mylonakis, E. MRSA Colonization and Risk of Infection in the Neonatal and Pediatric ICU: A Meta-Analysis. *Pediatrics.*, 2014, 133(4), 1015–23. doi:10.1542/peds.2013-3413.

[52] Boucher, HW; Corey, GR. Epidemiology of Methicillin-Resistant *Staphylococcus aureus*. *Clin Infect Dis.*, 2008, 46(5), S344–49. doi:10.1086/533590.

[53] Weeks, JL; Garcia-Prats, JA; Baker, CJ. Methicillin-Resistant *Staphylococcus aureus* Osteomyelitis in a Neonate. *JAMA.*, 1981, 245(16), 1662–64.

[54] Pinter, DM; Mandel, J; Hulten, KG; Minkoff, H; Tosi, MF. Maternal-Infant Perinatal Transmission of Methicillin-Resistant and Methicillin-

Sensitive *Staphylococcus aureus*. *Am J Perinatol.*, 2009, 26(2), 145–51. doi:10.1055/s-0028-1095179.

[55] Shiojima, T; Ohki, Y; Nako, Y; Morikawa, A; Okubo, T; Iyobe, S. Immediate Control of a Methicillin-Resistant *Staphylococcus aureus* Outbreak in a Neonatal Intensive Care Unit. *J Infect Chemother.*, 2003, 9(3), 243–47. doi:10.1007/s10156-003-0255-5.

[56] Huang, YC; Chou, YH; Su, LH; Lien, RI; Lin, TY. Methicillin-Resistant *Staphylococcus aureus* Colonization and Its Association with Infection among Infants Hospitalized in Neonatal Intensive Care Units. *Pediatrics.*, 2006, 118(2), 469–74. doi:10.1542/peds.2006-0254.

[57] Pimentel, JD; Meier, FA; Samuel, LP. Chorioamnionitis and Neonatal Sepsis from Community-Associated MRSA. *Emerging Infect Dis.*, 2009, 15(12), 2069–71. doi:10.3201/eid1512.090853.

[58] Behari, P; Englund, J; Alcasid, G; Garcia-Houchins, S; Weber, SG. Transmission of Methicillin-Resistant *Staphylococcus aureus* to Preterm Infants through Breast Milk. *Infect Control Hosp Epidemiol.*, 2004, 25(9), 778–80. doi:10.1086/502476.

[59] Gastelum, DT; Dassey, D; Mascola, L; Yasuda, LM. Transmission of Community-Associated Methicillin-Resistant *Staphylococcus aureus* from Breast Milk in the Neonatal Intensive Care Unit. *Pediatr Infect Dis J.*, 2005, 24(12), 1122–24.

[60] Filius, P; Margreet G; Gyssens, IC; Kershof, IM; Roovers, PJE; Ott, A; Vulto, AG; Verbrugh, HA; Endtz, HP. Colonization and Resistance Dynamics of Gram-Negative Bacteria in Patients during and after Hospitalization. *Antimicrob Agents Chemother.*, 2005, 49(7), 2879–86. doi:10.1128/AAC.49.7.2879-2886.2005.

[61] Lessa, FC; Edwards, JR; Fridkin, SK; Tenover, FC; Horan, TC; Gorwitz, RJ. Trends in Incidence of Late-Onset Methicillin-Resistant *Staphylococcus aureus* Infection in Neonatal Intensive Care Units: Data from the National Nosocomial Infections Surveillance System, 1995-2004. *Pediatr Infect Dis J.*, 2009, 28(7), 577–81. doi:10.1097/INF.0b013e31819988bf.

[62] Carey, AJ; Saiman, L; Polin, RA. Hospital-Acquired Infections in the NICU: Epidemiology for the New Millennium. *Clin Perinatol.*, 2008, 35(1), 223–49, x. doi:10.1016/j.clp.2007.11.014.

[63] Woodlief, RS; Markowitz, JE. Unrecognized Invasive Infection in a Neonate Colonized with Methicillin-Resistant *Staphylococcus aureus*. *J Pediatr.*, 2009, 155(6), 943–943.e1. doi:10.1016/j.jpeds.2009.07.025.

[64] Cimolai, N. *Staphylococcus aureus* Outbreaks among Newborns: New Frontiers in an Old Dilemma. *Am J Perinatol.*, 2003, 20(3), 125–36. doi:10.1055/s-2003-40010.

[65] Bizzarro, MJ; Gallagher, PG. Antibiotic-Resistant Organisms in the Neonatal Intensive Care Unit. *Semin Perinatol.*, 2007, 31(1), 26–32. doi:10.1053/j.semperi.2007.01.004.

[66] Gerber, SI; Jones, RC; Scott, MV; Price, JS; Dworkin, MS; Filippell, MB; Rearick, T; et al. Management of Outbreaks of Methicillin-Resistant *Staphylococcus aureus* Infection in the Neonatal Intensive Care Unit: A Consensus Statement. *Infect Control Hosp Epidemiol.*, 2006, 27(2), 139–45. doi:10.1086/501216.

[67] Saiman, L; Cronquist, A; Wu, F; Zhou, J; Rubenstein, D; Eisner, W; Kreiswirth, BN; Della-Latta, P. An Outbreak of Methicillin-Resistant *Staphylococcus aureus* in a Neonatal Intensive Care Unit. *Infect Control Hosp Epidemiol.*, 2003, 24(5), 317–21. doi:10.1086/502217.

[68] Eveillard, M; Martin, Y; Hidri, N; Boussougant, Y; Joly-Guillou, ML. Carriage of Methicillin-Resistant *Staphylococcus aureus* among Hospital Employees: Prevalence, Duration, and Transmission to Households. *Infect Control Hosp Epidemiol.*, 2004, 25(2), 114–20. doi:10.1086/502360.

[69] Carey, AJ; Duchon, J; Della-Latta, P; Saiman, L. The Epidemiology of Methicillin-Susceptible and Methicillin-Resistant *Staphylococcus aureus* in a Neonatal Intensive Care Unit, 2000-2007. *J Perinatol.*, 2010, 30(2), 135–39. doi:10.1038/jp.2009.119.

[70] Sakaki, H; Nishioka, M; Kanda, K; Takahashi, Y. An Investigation of the Risk Factors for Infection with Methicillin-Resistant *Staphylococcus aureus* among Patients in a Neonatal Intensive Care Unit. *Am J Infect Control.*, 2009, 37(7), 580–86. doi:10.1016/j.ajic.2009.02.008.

[71] Khoury, J; Jones, M; Grim, A; Dunne, WM; Fraser, V. Eradication of Methicillin-Resistant *Staphylococcus aureus* from a Neonatal Intensive Care Unit by Active Surveillance and Aggressive Infection Control Measures. *Infect Control Hosp Epidemiol.*, 2005, 26(7), 616–21. doi:10.1086/502590.

[72] Ziakas, PD; Anagnostou, T; Mylonakis, E. The Prevalence and Significance of Methicillin-Resistant *Staphylococcus aureus* Colonization at Admission in the General ICU Setting: A Meta-Analysis of Published Studies. *Crit Care Med.*, 2014, 42(2), 433–44. doi:10.1097/CCM.0b013e3182a66bb8.

[73] Macnow, T; O'Toole, D; DeLaMora, P; Murray, M; Rivera, K; Whittier, S; Ross, B; Jenkins, S; Saiman, L; Duchon, J. Utility of Surveillance Cultures for Antimicrobial Resistant Organisms in Infants Transferred to the Neonatal Intensive Care Unit. *Pediatr Infect Dis J.*, 2013, 32(12), 443–50. doi:10.1097/INF.0b013e3182a1d77f.

[74] Gregory, ML; Eichenwald, EC; Puopolo, KM. Seven-Year Experience with a Surveillance Program to Reduce Methicillin-Resistant *Staphylococcus aureus* Colonization in a Neonatal Intensive Care Unit. *Pediatrics.*, 2009, 123(5), 790–96. doi:10.1542/peds.2008-1526.

[75] Morioka, I; Yahata, M; Shibata, M; Miwa, A; Yokota, T; Jikimoto, T; Nakamura, M; et al. Impact of Pre-Emptive Contact Precautions for Outborn Neonates on the Incidence of Healthcare-Associated Meticillin-Resistant *Staphylococcus aureus* Transmission in a Japanese Neonatal Intensive Care Unit. *J Hosp Infect.*, 2013, 84(1), 66–70. doi:10.1016/j.jhin.2012.12.016.

[76] Kim, YH; Chang, SS; Kim, YS; Kim, EAR; Yun, SC; Kim, KS; Pi, SY. Clinical Outcomes in Methicillin-Resistant *Staphylococcus aureus* Colonized Neonates in the Neonatal Intensive Care Unit. *Neonatology.*, 2007, 91(4), 241–47. doi:10.1159/000098171.

[77] Maraqa, NF; Aigbivbalu, L; Masnita-Iusan, C; Wludyka, P; Shareef, Z; Bailey, C; Rathore, MH. Prevalence of and Risk Factors for Methicillin-Resistant *Staphylococcus aureus* Colonization and Infection among Infants at a Level III Neonatal Intensive Care Unit. *Am J Infect Control.*, 2011, 39(1), 35–41. doi:10.1016/j.ajic.2010.07.013.

[78] Gastmeier, P; Schwab, F; Bärwolff, S; Rüden, H; Grundmann, H. Correlation between the Genetic Diversity of Nosocomial Pathogens and Their Survival Time in Intensive Care Units. *J Hosp Infect.*, 2006, 62(2), 181–86. doi:10.1016/j.jhin.2005.08.010.

[79] Lin, YC; Lauderdale, TL; Lin, HM; Chen, PC; Cheng, MF; Hsieh, KS; Liu, YC. An Outbreak of Methicillin-Resistant *Staphylococcus aureus* Infection in Patients of a Pediatric Intensive Care Unit and High Carriage Rate among Health Care Workers. *J Microbiol Immunol Infect.*, 2007, 40(4), 325–34.

[80] Lawes, T; Edwards, B; López-Lozano, JM; Gould, I. Trends in *Staphylococcus aureus* Bacteraemia and Impacts of Infection Control Practices Including Universal MRSA Admission Screening in a Hospital in Scotland, 2006-2010: Retrospective Cohort Study and Time-Series Intervention Analysis. *BMJ Open.*, 2012, 2(3), doi:10.1136/bmjopen-2011-000797.

[81] Geraci, DM; Giuffrè, M; Bonura, C; Matranga, D; Aleo, A; Saporito, L; Corsello, G; Larsen, AR; Mammina, C. Methicillin-Resistant *Staphylococcus aureus* Colonization: A Three-Year Prospective Study in a Neonatal Intensive Care Unit in Italy. Edited by Paul J. Planet. *PLoS ONE.*, 9 2014, (2) e87760. doi:10.1371/journal.pone.0087760.

*Chapter 7*

# STAPHYLOCOCCUS SPP. IN THE ETIOLOGY OF PERITONITIS IN PERITONEAL DIALYSIS: RISK FACTORS OF THE HOST AND MICROORGANISM

*Ana Cláudia Moro Lima dos Santos*
*and Maria de Lourdes Ribeiro de Souza da Cunha*[*]
Department of Microbiology and Immunology, Botucatu Institute of
Biosciences, UNESP - Univ Estadual Paulista,
Botucatu, São Paulo State, Brazil

## ABSTRACT

Bacterial peritonitis remains a major complication of peritoneal dialysis (PD), often leading to the interruption of the technique and an important impact on mortality. When such episodes are serious and long, they may lead to lesion of the peritoneal membrane. Therefore, PD professionals highlight the prevention and treatment of these infections aiming at a quick resolution, which contributes to the preservation of the peritoneal membrane function. The clinical presentation and progression of the episode of peritonitis are significantly influenced by characteristics of the causative agent. PD peritonitis is in most cases caused by Gram-positive cocci - *Staphylococcus* spp. – including the species of

---
[*] Corresponding author: cunhamlr@ibb.unesp.br

Coagulase-negative staphylococci (CoNS) and *S. aureus*. The CoNS group comprises more than 50 species, and some of them are already well established as causes of PD-related peritonitis, especially *S. epidermidis*. In general, peritonitis caused by CoNS shows a light clinical course and has a high rate of resolution, but recurrent infections that had apparently been cured are observed. *S. aureus* is associated with: more severe episodes, a worse overall prognosis compared to other peritonitis, a higher risk of hospitalization, catheter removal, and death, while these patients are significantly more likely to switch to hemodialysis. The severity of *S. aureus* infections is associated with virulence factors produced by these bacteria, such as enzymes and several toxins with various activities including those which damage cell membranes and which function as superantigens. Another important virulence factor for the occurrence of peritonitis is biofilm production by *S. aureus* and mainly by CoNS, which facilitates bacterial adhesion to catheters and colonization of the infection site, and protects the bacterial cells from natural defense mechanisms and from antibiotic action. The treatment of these infections can also be unsuccessful due to the presence of resistance genes that these microorganisms may have, i.e., the presence of *mecA* gene that causes methicillin resistance. This gene is located in a mobile genetic element called staphylococcal cassette chromosome *mec* (SCC*mec*) which allows transmission of the resistance characteristic with important implications as it results in limiting the use of β-lactam antibiotics. One of the contributing factors for infections caused by *S. aureus* is the fact that PD patients are more likely to be nasal carriers of *S. aureus* when compared to the healthy population, and then it is an important risk factor for infections. Studies using typing methods have shown that the nasal isolate from the carrier and the strain causing the peritonitis are often indistinguishable. Thus, there has been a significant decrease in the rates of infections by *S. aureus* in recent years with the use of topical antibiotics for decolonization, especially mupirocin. Therefore, this chapter aims at addressing issues related to PD peritonitis caused by *Staphylococcus* spp. highlighting the epidemiology and risk factors of the host and microorganism when these infections occur.

# INTRODUCTION

Peritoneal Dialysis (PD) is one of the main treatment modalities for patients with renal insufficiency in the final stage. Peritoneal infection remains the major complication of this technique, which often causes withdrawal and an important impact on mortality. The mortality of PD patients is about 18% despite a series of technological innovations that have reduced overall infection rates over the past decades [1].When these episodes are severe and prolonged, they can lead to lesions on the peritoneal membrane, which makes the technique impracticable and promotes change for hemodialysis. Therefore, the support staff of DP aims at the prevention and treatment of these infections seeking a quick resolution that contributes to the preservation of the function of the peritoneal membrane [2-3].

The clinical presentation and progression of the peritonitis episode are significantly influenced by the characteristics of the etiological agent, which is a definitive marker of mortality. The patient's demographic factors such as age, gender, nutrition, and diabetes mellitus are also significant in the outcome these infections [4].

PD peritonitis are caused in most episodes by Gram-positive cocci, especially *Staphylococcus* spp. including Coagulase-negative Staphylococci (CoNS), etiologically predominant, followed by *Staphylococcus aureus* [2, 5]. The CoNS group comprises more than 50 species [6], among which some are already known to cause infections related to DP, especially *S. epidermidis*. In general, peritonitis caused by CoNS has a mild clinical course and a high rate of resolution [7]. However, there is recurrence of seemingly healed infections. *S. aureus* is associated with more severe episodes and poorer overall prognosis compared to other peritonitis, with increased risk of hospitalization, catheter removal, and death; besides, these patients are significantly more likely to switching treatments, such as to hemodialysis.

## VIRULENCE FACTORS

The severity of *S. aureus* infections is associated with virulence factors produced by these bacteria, such as enzymes and several toxins with various activities, including toxins that damage cell membranes and the superantigens [8]. Some of the enzymes produced are: coagulase, which acts on fibrinogen converting it into fibrin. Such enzyme is important for the pathogenesis of the staphylococcal infection as it protects the microorganism by forming a clot around the site of infection, causing it to be unidentified by the immune system and thus remain intact inside; staphylokinase, which is capable of dissolving fibrin and allowing fluidization of clots and the mobilization of the pathogen; hyaluronidase and lipases, which are enzymes that degrade connective tissues with infiltration of host bacteria and spread; and penicillinase, which grant resistance to the antimicrobials whose active compound is penicillin [9].

The staphylococcal toxins produced by *S. aureus* and CoNS are potent in damaging the human body and can be generally divided into two groups: membrane active agents including alpha, beta, delta, and gamma toxins and Panton-Valentine leukocidin; and toxins with superantigen activity including the group of pyrogenic toxin superantigens (PTSAgs). These toxins include the staphylococcal enterotoxins, toxic shock syndrome toxin 1 (TSST-1), and the family of exfoliative toxins [10]. The genes encoding these toxins are located on mobile genetic elements, such as phages and *S. aureus* pathogenic islands (SAPIs), which are potentially mobile DNA segments of variable length encoding genes associated with virulence and are horizontally transferred between strains [11].

Other important virulence factors for peritonitis to occur are biofilm production and the presence of resistance genes. The production of biofilm - an extracellular polysaccharide - by *S. aureus* and primarily by CoNS facilitates bacterial adherence to catheters and the colonization of the infection site. This protects the bacterial cells from the natural defense mechanisms and from the antibiotic action directly and prevents the presence of such penetration agents of the bacterial cell, or indirectly by maintaining the cell in a quiescent state. For these reasons, biofilm formation is considered to be the main virulence factor of CoNS [10].

## CHARACTERISTICS OF THE PATHOGEN AND THE HOST IN THE EVOLUTION OF PERITONITIS

The treatment of these infections can also be unsuccessful due to the presence of resistance genes in these microorganisms, such as the *mecA* gene, which grants resistance to methicillin. This gene is located in a mobile genetic element called staphylococcal cassette chromosome *mec* (*SCCmec*) that allows the transmission of the resistance characteristic with important implications for it results in limiting the use of beta-lactam antibiotics [3, 12].

Some studies have compared the clinical course of infections caused by such species in recent years in order to determine the progressively increasing resistance rates observed among the CoNS and the impact of this increase in outcomes and complications of infections caused by these organisms.

A research group from the Dialysis Unit at the Clinical Hospital of Botucatu Medical School (HC-FMB) conducted several studies involving patients undergoing Continuous Ambulatory Peritoneal Dialysis (CAPD) in order to describe the microbiological properties of the staphylococci causing peritonitis, and made comparisons with *S. aureus* infections. Thus, associations between the characteristics of the pathogen and the host were established in the evolution of these infections.

In 2005, a study carried out from 1996 to 2000 showed that the peritonitis resolution was not influenced by the host factors (age, gender, diabetes, use of vancomycin, exchange system, or dialysis duration), whereas the etiology *S. aureus* was independently associated with an outcome worse than the episodes caused by CoNS [13], as previously demonstrated. Factors related to the species and antimicrobial resistance could explain these results. Resistance to oxacillin is more frequent among CoNS than in *S. aureus*. However, there was no difference in the resolution rate between the strains resistant and susceptible to oxacillin, so the contribution of the antimicrobial resistance was inconsistent to explain worse outcomes. The results of this study suggest that the virulence factors most often found in *S. aureus* accounted for a more aggressive nature of the infection and a consequent worse outcome.

In 2009, a publication of such research group using two logistic regression models supported this hypothesis. In the first model that does not include virulence factors, the resolution probability was not influenced by the host factors, but it was higher for the episodes caused by *S. epidermidis* compared with *S. aureus*. In contrast, using the second model including virulence factors, no difference was observed in the resolution probability between the episodes of *S. aureus* and *S. epidermidis* peritonitis. This result can be explained by the fact that including enzymes and toxins in the model allowed the effect of these factors on the species to be controlled. The effect observed in the first model of episodes by *S. aureus* may be due to the effect of pathogenicity factors that are more common in this species. In addition, the second model of episodes caused by *S. epidermidis* showed a resolution rate lower than for those caused by other species of CoNS, regardless the virulence factors [14]. Some recent studies describe *S. epidermidis* as a versatile organism that can live as a commensal and pathogenic bacterium. Moreover, this species uses sophisticated mechanisms of gene regulation to quickly adapt its metabolism in response to changes in the external environment, to communicate with other cells in the ecological niche, and to escape from the host immune response [15]. These results highlight the importance of the exact identification of the species of CoNS because they behave differently and should not be evaluated as a group but rather as distinct species with specific characteristics which can cause severe infections like *S. schleiferi, S. lugdunensis, S. warneri,* and helps distinguish the contaminated cultures from the true infections. The clinical approach to be adopted should be appropriate for each species, although many routine laboratories still do not identify the CoNS species because of their difficult identification. This has become possible due to automated and fast systems, and the MALDI-TOF (Matrix Assisted Leisure Desorption Ionization - Time o Flight) stands out for the best performance [16]. Even though there are around 20 clinically relevant species of CoNS, these are sometimes difficult to identify even by automated systems, and hence require a molecular approach by sequencing the DNA encoding 16S rRNA.

In 2011, an analysis of 115 episodes of peritonitis by CoNS that occurred in 74 patients between 1994 and 2011 at this university center was conducted, and it aimed to evaluate the production of biofilms, enzymes, and toxins. The results showed that oxacillin susceptibility and vancomycin use as the first treatment were the only independent predictors of resolution, which reinforces the validity of the International Society of Peritoneal Dialysis (ISPD) guidelines on the monitoring of bacterial resistance so as to set initial treatment protocols. Such results also suggest that the presence of biofilm is a potential cause of repeated episodes of peritonitis [17].

Also in 2011, a study was carried out with 62 episodes of peritonitis caused by *S. aureus* between 1996 and 2010 in order to identify bacterial factors that influenced the outcome of peritonitis through the production of biofilm, enzymes, toxins, and oxacillin resistance based on the minimum inhibitory concentration and presence of the *mecA* gene. The results showed that the production of toxins and enzymes was significant, except for the enterotoxin D production. Biofilm production was positive in 88.7% of the strains, and the presence of the *mecA* gene was associated with a higher frequency of fever and abdominal pain.There was a trend of higher mortality rate for the episodes of *S. aureus* (9.7%) compared with the episodes by CoNS (2.5%) ($p = 0.08$), while the resolution rates were similar. The result of this infection was negatively influenced by host factors such as age and diabetes mellitus. Furthermore, the production of beta-hemolysin was a predictive factor for the no resolution of the infection, which suggests a pathogenic role of this factor in PD-related *S. aureus* peritonitis [18]. The production of α-hemolysin was also related to the worse evolution of peritonitis in a previous study, with a resolution rate of 8.2 times higher for peritonitis caused by *Staphylococcus* spp. that did not produce this toxin [14]. These results corroborate the data published by Haslinger-Löffler et al. [19] suggesting that α-hemolysin plays a specific role in the peritonitis pathogenesis. These authors showed that only invasive and α-hemolysin producers *S. aureus* induced the death of caspase-independent mesothelial cells. Unlike *S. aureus*, cytotoxic effects of *S. epidermidis* strains tested that were not invasive and did not produce α-hemolysin were not observed. Such results indicate that α-hemolysin and beta-hemolysin are important mechanisms of *S. aureus* to cause persistent damage to the peritoneum during peritonitis.

Another contributing factor for *S. aureus* infections is the fact that PD patients are more likely to be nasal carriers of *S. aureus* compared to the healthy population, which is an important risk factor for infections - both of exit site infections (ESI) and of peritonitis. Some studies using typing methods demonstrated that carrier's nasal isolated and the strain causing peritonitis are often indistinguishable [20]. Therefore, the eradication of this type of carriage proved necessary. The effect of intermittent *S. aureus* eradication on the infection rates with the use of topical antibiotics for decolonization was then assessed. Thus, *S. aureus* infection rates have shown significant reduction, especially with the use of mupirocin. The nasal mupirocin effect was evaluated by a study in which a control group was compared with a cohort treated prospectively. This showed a statistically significant reduction in the infections of the treated group and also an increase in the rate of these infections by gram-negative bacteria. In a prospective randomized placebo controlled clinical trial for nasal mupirocin, a significant reduction in the rate of *S. aureus* ESI was reported, but a reduced rate of *S. aureus* peritonitis was not statistically significant. The effect of topical mupirocin applied to the exit site was also evaluated by a prospective controlled study in which both indices of ESI and *S. aureus* peritonitis were significantly reduced. Together, these studies indicate that infection rates can be reduced by the intermittent carriage eradication, but it may not prevent all cases [21-26].

## THERAPY

Besides the use of mupirocin and for all evidence described above, there is a need to develop effective measures in clinical practice against infections caused by CoNS and *S.aureus*. In this sense, ISPD– through the results already presented in some studies – brings some considerations and recommendations. Regarding CoNS infections, these generally have a mild form of peritonitis and promptly respond to antibiotic therapy. Relapse often occurs due to biofilm formation; under such circumstance, the catheter should be replaced [26-29]. Depending on the species involved, there is a very high rate of methicillin resistance (> 50%); therefore, vancomycin is used as empiric therapy. Such resistance must be established based on the levels of Minimum

Inhibitory Concentration (MIC) and ideally by molecular data (e.g., the presence of *mecA* gene). Every effort should be made to avoid inadequate levels of antibiotics that can lead to relapse of peritonitis. Ideally, the cell counts and effluent cultures should guide the therapy, and a two-week treatment is usually enough.

Peritonitis caused by *S. aureus*, which is responsible for severe peritonitis, is unlikely to respond to antibiotic therapy without catheter removal if it is concomitant with tunnel or exit-site infection [30-32], and the patient can be introduced into the technique again after a rest period off PD of usually a minimum of 2 weeks. The use of 600 mg/day of rifampicin orally (in single or divided doses) may be added to the intraperitoneal antibiotics as an auxiliary for relapse or repetitive peritonitis prevention, but the inducing effect of rifampicin drug-metabolizing enzymes, which reduces the serum levels of many drugs, should be considered in patients taking other medications [33]. Therapy with this adjuvant antibiotic should be limited to a week since resistance occurs over long periods of treatment. Moreover, if the patient has a high risk of having asymptomatic tuberculosis, rifampicin should be used carefully in order to preserve this drug for the tuberculosis treatment.

As in CoNS infections, patients should be treated with vancomycin if the *S. aureus* strain is methicillin resistant, and these infections are more difficult to resolve when compared with methicillin-sensitive *S. aureus* peritonitis. Vancomycin may be administered intraperitoneally (IP) as 15-30 mg/kg of body weight with a maximum dose of 2g. A typical protocol for a patient of 50-60 kg is 1g vancomycin IP every 5 days. Ideally, the repetitive dosing period should be based on minimum levels and is likely to be every 3-5 days. The dosage range depends on the residual kidney function, and the patients should receive another dose when serum levels reach 15 mg/ml. Teicoplanin, when available, can be used at a dose of 15 mg/kg bodyweight every 5-7 days. Data for children suggest that this approach is successful for both CAPD and APD, and the treatment should last 3 weeks [34, 35].

In a recent review of 245 cases of *S. aureus* peritonitis, episodes that were initially treated with vancomycin had a better initial response rate than those who were treated with cefazolin (98.0% vs. 85.2%, p = 0.001), but complete healing rate was similar [33]. Rifampicing-adjuvant treatment for a period of 5-7 days was associated with a significantly lower risk of relapse or recurrence of *S. aureus* peritonitis when compared to what occurred in the treatment without rifampicin (21.4% vs. 42.8%). In this study, hospitalization was an important risk factor in cases of methicillin resistance. Similarly, a review of 503 cases of staphylococcal peritonitis in Australia revealed that the initial empiric antibiotic choice between vancomycin and cefazolin was not associated with any significant differences in subsequent clinical outcomes [36]. Unfortunately, prolonged vancomycin therapy may predispose PD patients to vancomycin-resistant *S. aureus* infections, which should be avoided whenever possible, but if it occurs, other antibiotics such as linezolid, daptomycin, or quinupristin/dalfopristin may be used.

## REFERENCES

[1] Tolkoff-Rubin, NE; Varma, P; Rubin, RH. Infections in peritoneal dialysis. In: Sweny, P; Rubin, R;Tolkoff-Rubin, N; eds. *The Infectious Complications of Renal Disease*. Oxford, UK: Oxford University Press; 2003, 153–75.

[2] Davenport, A. Peritonitis remains the major clinical complication of peritoneal dialysis: the London, UK, peritonitis audit 2002-2003. *Perit Dial Int.*, 2009, 29 (3), 297-302.

[3] Li, PK; Szeto, CC; Piraino, B; Bernardini, J; Figueiredo, AE; Gupta, A; Johnson, DW; Kuijper, EJ; Lye, WC; Salzer, W; Schaefer, F; Struijk, DG. International Society for Peritoneal Dialysis. *Perit Dial Int.*, 2010, 30(4), 393-423

[4] Pérez Fontan, M; Rodríguez-Carmona, A; García-Naveiro, R; Rosales, M; Villaverde, P; Valdés, F. Peritonitis-related mortality in patients undergoing chronic peritoneal dialysis. *Perit Dial Int.*, 2005, 25(3), 274-84.

[5] Mujais, S. Microbiology and outcomes of peritonitis in North America. *Kidney Int Suppl.*, 2006, 103, S55–62.

[6] Euzéby, JP. List of prokaryotic names with standing in nomenclature - genus *Staphylococcus*. Available at: http://www.bacterio.net/s/staphylococcus.html. Accessed May 10, 2016.

[7] Troidle, L; Gordban-Brennan, N; Kliger, A; Finkeltein, F. Differing outcomes of gram-positive and gram-negative. *Am J KidneyDis.*,1998, 32(4), 623-8.

[8] Ghali, JR; Bannister, KM; Brown, FG; Rosman, JB; Wiggins, KJ; Johnson, DW; McDonald, SP. Microbiology and outcomes of peritonitis in Australian peritoneal dialysis patients. *Perit Dial Int.*, 2011, 31(6), 651-62.

[9]  Murray, PR; Rosenthal, KS; Kobayashi, OS; Pfaller, MA. *Microbiologia Médica*. 4a ed. Rio de Janeiro: Guanabara Koogan, 2004.
[10] Bohach, GA; Fast, DJ; Nelson, RD; Schlievert, PM. Staphylococcal and streptococcal pyrogenic toxins involved in toxic shock syndrome and related illnesses. *Crit Rev Microbiol.*, 1990, 17(4), 251-72.
[11] Hanssen, AM; EricsonSollid, JU. SCC*mec* in staphylococci: genes on the move. *FEMS Immunol Med Microbiol.*, 2006, 46(1), 8-20.
[12] Martins, A; Cunha, ML. Methicillin resistance in *Staphylococcus aureus* and coagulase-negative staphylococci: Epidemiological and molecular aspects. *Microbiol Immunol.*, 2007, 51, 787–795.
[13] Cunha, MLRS; Montelli, AC; Fioravante, AM; Batalha, JEN; Caramori, JCT; Barretti, P. Predictive factors of outcome following staphylococcal peritonitis in continuous ambulatory peritoneal dialysis. *Clin Nephrol.*, 2005, 64(5), 378-82.
[14] Barretti, P; Montelli, AC; Batalha JEN; Caramori, JCT; Cunha, MLRS. The role of virulence factors in the outcome of staphylococcal peritonitis in CAPD patients. *BMC Infect Dis.*, 2009, 9, 212-9.
[15] Schoenfelder, SMK; Langea, S; Eckart, M; Hennig, S; Kozytska, S; Ziebuhr, W. Sucess through diversity – How *Staphylococcus epidermidis* establishes as a nosocomial pathogen. *Int J of Medical Microb.*, 2010, 300(6), 380-386.
[16] Dupont, C; Sivadon-Tardy, V; Bille, E; Dauphin, B; Beretti, J; Alvarez, A; et al. Identification of clinical coagulase negative staphylococci, isolated in microbiology laboratories, by matrix-assisted laser desorption/ionization-time of flight mass spectrometry and two automated systems. *Clin Microbiol Infect*. Epub 2 Sep 2009 as doi:10:1111/j.14690691.2009.03036.
[17] Camargo, CH; Cunha, MLRS; Caramori, JC; Mondelli, AL; Montelli, AC; Barretti, P. Peritoneal Dialysis–Related Peritonitis due to Coagulase-Negative *Staphylococcus*: A Review of 115 Cases in a Brazilian Center. *Clin J Am Soc Nephrol.*, 2014, 9(6), 1074–1081.
[18] Barretti, P; Moraes, TM; Camargo, CH; Caramori, JC; Mondelli, AL; Montelli, AC; Cunha, MLRS. Peritoneal dialysis-related peritonitis due to *Staphylococcus aureus*: a single-center experience over 15 years. *PLoS One.*, 2012, 7(2), e31780. doi: 10.1371/journal.pone.0031780. Epub 2012 Feb 21.

[19] Haslinger-Loffler, B; Wagner, B; Bruck, M; Strangfeld, K; Grundmeier, M; Fischer, U; Volker, W; Peters, G; Schulze-Osthoff, K; Sinha, B. *Staphylococcus aureus* induces caspase-independent cell death in human peritoneal mesothelial cells. *Kidney Int.* 2006, 70, 1089-1098.

[20] Peacock, SJ; Howe, PA; Day, NP; Crook, DW; Winearls, CG; Berendt, AR. Outcome following staphylococcal peritonitis. *Perit Dial Int.*, 2000, 20, 215–219.

[21] Zimakoff, J; Bangsgaard Pedersen, F; Bergen, L; Baago–Nielsen, J; Daldorph, B; Espersen, F; et al. *Staphylococcus aureus* carriage and infections among patients in four haemo- and peritoneal-dialysis centres in Denmark. *J Hosp Infect.*, 1996; 33, 289–300.

[22] Vandenbergh, MFQ; Verbrugh, HA. Carriage of *Staphylococcus aureus*: epidemiology and clinical relevance. *J Lab Clin Med.*, 1999, 133, 525–34.

[23] Herwaldt, LA. Reduction of *Staphylococcus aureus* nasal carriage and infection in dialysis patients. *J Hosp Infect.*, 1998, 40, S13–23.

[24] Perez–Fontan, M; Garcia–Falcon, T; Rosales, M; Rodriguez–Carmona, A; Adeva, M; Rodriguez–Lozano, L, et al. Treatment of *Staphylococcus aureus* carriers in continuous ambulatory peritoneal dialysis with mupirocin: long-term results. *Am J Kidney Dis.*, 1993, 22,708–12.

[25] Mupirocin Study Group. Nasal mupirocin prevents *Staphylococcus aureus* exit-site infection during peritoneal dialysis. *J Am Soc Nephrol.*, 1996, 28, 1898–902.

[26] Thodis, E; Bhaskaran, S; Pasadakis, P; Bargman, JM; Vas, SI; Oreopoulos, DG. Decrease in *Staphylococcus aureus* exit-site infections and peritonitis in CAPD patients by local application of mupirocin ointment at the catheter exit site. *Perit Dial Int.*, 1998; 18, 261–70.

[27] Swartz, R; Messana, J; Reynolds, J; Ranjit, U. Simultaneous catheter replacement and removal in refractory peritoneal dialysis infections. *Kidney Int.*, 1991, 40,1160–5.

[28] Finkelstein, ES; Jekel, J; Troidle, L; Gorban-Brennan, N; Finkelstein, FO; Bia, FJ. Patterns of infection in patients maintained on long-term peritoneal dialysis therapy with multiple episodes of peritonitis. *Am J Kidney Dis.*, 2002, 39, 1278–86.

[29] Dasgupta, MK; Ward, K; Noble, PA; Larabie, M; Costerton, JW. Development of bacterial biofilms on Silastic catheter materials in peritoneal dialysis fluid. *Am J Kidney Dis.*, 1994, 23, 709–16.

[30] Read, RR; Eberwein, P; Dasgupta, MK; Grant, SK; Lam, K; Nickel, JC; et al. Peritonitis in peritoneal dialysis: bacterial colonization by biofilm spread along the catheter surface. *Kidney Int.*, 1989, 35, 614–21.

[31] Bayston, R; Andrews, M; Rigg, K; Shelton, A. Recurrent infection and catheter loss in patients on continuous ambulatory peritoneal dialysis. *Perit Dial Int.*, 1999, 19:550–5

[32] Gupta, B; Bernardini, J; Piraino, B. Peritonitis associated with exit site and tunnel infections. *Am J Kidney Dis.*, 1996, 28, 415–19

[33] Lye, WC; Leong, SO; van der Straaten, J; Lee, EJ. *Staphylococcus aureus* CAPD-related infections are associated with nasal carriage. *Adv Perit Dial.*, 1994, 10, 163–5.

[34] Szeto, CC; Chow, KM; Kwan, BC; Law, MC; Chung, KY; Yu, S; et al. *Staphylococcus aureus* peritonitis complicates peritoneal dialysis: review of 245 consecutive cases. *Clin J Am Soc Nephrol.*, 2007, 2, 245–51.

[35] Manley, HJ; McClaran, ML; Bedenbaugh, A; Peloquin, CA. Linezolid stability in peritoneal dialysis solutions. *Perit Dial Int.*, 2002, 22,419–22

[36] Govindarajulu, S; Hawley, CM; McDonald, SP; Brown, FG; Rosman, JB; Wiggins, KJ; et al. *Staphylococcus aureus* peritonitis in Australian peritoneal dialysis patients: predictors, treatment and outcomes in 503 cases. *Perit Dial Int.*, 2010, 30,311–19. Epub 26 Feb 2010 as doi:10.3747/pdi. 2008.00258.

In: *Staphylococcus aureus*
Editor: M. L. R. S. Cunha

ISBN: 978-1-63485-959-2
© 2017 Nova Science Publishers, Inc.

*Chapter 8*

# *STAPHYLOCOCCUS AUREUS*: SUPERANTIGENS AND AUTOIMMUNITY

## *Thais Graziela Donegá França and Maria de Lourdes Ribeiro de Souza da Cunha*[*]

Department of Microbiology and Immunology, Botucatu Institute of Biosciences, UNESP - Univ Estadual Paulista. Botucatu, São Paulo State, Brazil

### ABSTRACT

*Staphylococcus aureus* is one of the most prevalent pathogens in the human population. *S. aureus* exhibits several escape mechanisms that allow it to evade host defenses. The main evasion mechanisms include inhibition of neutrophil chemotaxis; release of toxins that kill leukocytes; resistance to phagocytosis, complement system inactivation and production of several toxins defined as superantigens (SAgs). These toxins can activate a high proportion of T cells due to their ability to bind to both MHC class II molecules in antigen presenting cells and specific Vβ regions in the T cell receptor. This activation results in the polyclonal stimulation of T cells and an elevated production of proinflammatory cytokines. Bacterial superantigens are potent T cell activators that can activate T cells with specificity for antigens of the central nervous system. Experimental and epidemiological evidence support the theory that *S. aureus* that produces SAgs may be implicated in the genesis of

---

[*] Corresponding author: cunhamlr@ibb.unesp.br

Multiple sclerosis, septic arthritis, lupus and others autoimmune diseases. Multiple sclerosis is a demyelinating disease of the central nervous system, which is mainly mediated by T cells that are specific for the myelin self-antigen. These auto reactive T cells are generated in the periphery and cross the blood-brain barrier to the brain parenchyma where they initiate an autoimmune attack on the myelin sheath. Infectious disease agents can modulate autoimmune diseases in many different ways, such as triggering these pathologies or, contrarily, preventing their development. This chapter aims to describe about staphylococcal superantigens and the effect SAgs in the development of autoimmune diseases.

# INTRODUCTION

*Staphylococcus aureus* is a Gram-positive bacterium commonly found on the skin and mucous membranes of humans and animals [1]. Approximately 20-60% of the human population has nose mucosa colonized by this bacterium asymptomatically [2, 3]. Although *S. aureus* can asymptomatically colonize healthy people, it can also show pathogenic behavior.

*S. aureus* causes a variety of infectious diseases, for example, superficial skin infections and infections resulting in severe life threatening diseases, such as sepsis, pneumonia, and meningitis [4, 5]. The bacterium poses a serious public health problem in both hospitals and communities. The emergence of strains that are resistant to methicillin (MRSA) has increased the risk of spreading infectious diseases caused by *S. aureus*. Studies have demonstrated the contribution of MRSA strains in the development of several pathologies [6, 7, 8].

The skin acts as a barrier to the entry of microorganisms through a series of immunological, specific, and nonspecific mechanisms. *S. aureus* exhibits several escape mechanisms that allow it to evade host defenses. The main evasion mechanisms include inhibition of neutrophil chemotaxis [9]; release of toxins that kill leukocytes [10]; resistance to phagocytosis [11]; and complement system inactivation [12]. In addition, several enterotoxins are described (A, B, C, D, E, G, H, I, J, K, L, M, N, O, P, Q, R, S, T, U, V, X, and toxin1 of toxic-shock syndrome – TSST-1) which are defined as superantigens [13, 14, 15].

## SUPERANTIGENS

The superantigens (SAgs) were first found in the species *S. aureus* and *Streptococcus pyogenes*, and they have recently been described in newly discovered species as *Staphylococcus* coagulase-negative, *Mycoplasma arthritidis*, and *Yersinia pseudotuberculosis* [15]. These bacterial SAgs are able to stimulate a large number of T cells, regardless of their specificities [16, 17].

Triggering of the immune response by these superantigenic molecules differs from conventional antigens in several aspects. For instance, conventional antigens are initially processed such that peptides are generated. These peptides bind to histocompatibility molecules (MHC) of class I or class II, and such complexes are presented to the specific T lymphocytes. T lymphocytes, in turn, use the variable region of their antigen receptors (TCR) to recognize the association between peptide and MHC. Conversely, SAgs remain as intact molecules and bind directly to the MHC class II molecules exposed on the surface of the antigen presenting cells (APCs), without prior processing [18]. SAgs bind to class II molecules at a site distinct from that in which the conventional antigen peptide binds [19]. This SAg/MHC II complex interacts directly with the variable region of the β chain (vβ) of the TCR, determining the activation of APCs and lymphocytes [15, 3]. This triggered immune response during pathogenic invasion can lead to the breakdown of homeostasis between cell (Th1) and humoral (Th2) immunity, initiating the development of autoimmune diseases or aggravating existing symptoms [20, 21, 22].

Epidemiological and experimental evidence supports the theory that infectious agents, such as *S. aureus* and its products, the superantigens, are directly related to the development or exacerbation of autoimmune diseases, such as multiple sclerosis [23, 14, 24]. Multiple sclerosis is a demyelinating disease of the central nervous system, and it is mediated by specific T cells against myelin. These autoreactive T cells are peripheral and cross the blood brain barrier initiating the inflammatory process in the healthy myelin sheath.

Mehrabi and Asgari [24] demonstrated that *S. aureus* had higher prevalence in nasal swab samples from patients with multiple sclerosis in remission and relapse phase than healthy individuals. These rates were 50%, 68.3%, and 23.7%, respectively. They also noted that the group of patients with recurrence of the disease exhibited higher resistance to antibiotics. Similar results were observed in another study in Canada, which demonstrated that patients in both the relapse phase of the disease and in the remission phase showed similar rates of colonization in the nostrils. The rates were 21.2% and 27.3%, respectively. Importantly, these researchers showed that multiple sclerosis patients colonized with *S. aureus* are more susceptible to disease exacerbation than non colonized patients [14].

In this context, enterotoxin B (SEB) and TSST-1 are the bacterial superantigens best described in the literature associated with autoimmune diseases. SEB consists of a single polypeptide of 28000 Da coiled in the form of two domains [25]. This enterotoxin is highly resistant to cleavage by proteases due to its very compact tertiary structure. In terms of interaction with T cells, SEB recognizes the following subclasses of v$\beta$ humans: v$\beta$ 3, 12, 13.2, 14, 15, 17, and 20 [26].

Argudín et al. [27] demonstrated that SEB can penetrate the intestinal wall, initiating the absorption of water and electrolytes, thereby inducing local and systemic immune responses. Plaza et al. [28] confirmed that administration of SEB *in vivo* induces an exaggerated immune response, characterized by the release of Th1-type cytokines, as well as IL-2, IFN-$\gamma$ and IL-12 after 48–72h. Laouini et al. [29] showed that exposure to SEB induced production of IL-4 but not secretion of IFN-$\gamma$ on the skin of BALB/c mice. SEB is classically associated with food poisoning, but recently, it has been shown that SEB can initiate an increased systemic activation of the immune system, causing the development of autoimmune diseases such as multiple sclerosis, lupus, and rheumatoid arthritis [30].

## AUTOIMMUNE DISEASES

The role of enterotoxin B in multiple sclerosis is unknown, but it is involved in the reactivation of experimental autoimmune encephalitis (EAE) in mice and rats. Some studies have shown that SEB is responsible not only for the aggravation of the disease, but that it also contributes to the early development of EAE in PL/J mice by activation of T v$\beta$8 cells [23, 31]. Racke et al. [32], however, observed that T v$\beta$8 mice cells specific for myelin were unable to induce the disease when restimulated *in vitro*. Similar results were observed when triggering the immune response with an expansion of autoreactive T cells induced by SEB. Soos et al. [33] observed that this might result in an overload of the immune system by inducing anergy stage in the cells or by inducing apoptosis. Thus, these researchers demonstrated that PL/J mice infected with SEB did not develop EAE.

Lupus is a chronic inflammatory autoimmune disease that affects multiple organs. This disease is characterized by polyclonal B cell activation with production of high levels of autoantibodies. Genetic and environmental factors contribute to the development of this autoimmune disease, for example, hormone deregulation occurrence at puberty, specific drugs or viral infections [8].

The literature reaches no consensus on the influence of SEB in lupus development. The hypothesis in which SEB influences the course or development of lupus was suggested by Chowdhary et al. [34]. These researchers demonstrated that chronic exposure to small concentrations of SEB resulted in a chronic multisystem inflammatory disease in HLA-DQ8 transgenic mice. This experiment resulted in increased levels of anti-dsDNA and anti-Sm, T-lymphocyte infiltration in the liver and kidney, significant expansion of CD4 + Foxp3 +, as well as the increase of T cell receptors vβ8 + Foxp3 + Tregs in mice spleen. Kim et al. [35], however, suggested that SEB administration has a protective effect on lupus induction. SEB was able to reduce the disease in MRL/lpr mice by T vβ8 + cell reduction and T CD4- CDS-cells.

The effect of SEB in the development of autoimmune diseases always begins with the same principle, i.e., exacerbated activation of T vβ specific cells and B cells, causing a deregulation of the immune response. This effect was also observed in experimental models of rheumatoid arthritis (RA). Rheumatoid arthritis is an autoimmune disease characterized by inflammation and destruction of joints. Synovial histology fluid from RA patients showed elevated levels of IgM in serum for SEB when compared with healthy individuals [32, 36]. These results were confirmed by experimental studies for RA, and collagen-induced arthritis (CIA). SEB activated specific autoreactive T vβ8 cells and produced inflammatory cytokines such as IL-2 and IFN-γ, which are important mediators in causing destruction of joints [37].

The bacterial superantigen TSST-1 is also described in the literature as a potential agent in the development of infectious diseases and in the exacerbation of autoimmune diseases. This powerful SAg interacts with the subpopulation of T vβ cells 2 and 4, resulting in the most common cause of toxic shock syndrome (TSS). TSS is an acute and potentially fatal disease characterized by high fever, scaly diffuse rash, hypotension and the involvement of three or more organs [4, 15]. This toxin is produced by approximately 20% of the *S. aureus* samples isolated from human patients. A possible participation of TSST-1, SEA and SEB, has been described in autoimmune pathologies. These superantigens were able to reactivate experimental autoimmune encephalitis in mice [23, 31].

Stinssem et al. [38] showed that Tγδ cells from the cerebrospinal fluid and blood of patients with multiple sclerosis were reactivated in the presence of these superantigens when compared to healthy subjects. Reactivation of these cells caused cytotoxicity and brain injuries. Other researchers investigated the presence of *S. aureus* in the nostrils of patients with MS in remission phase, relapse phase, and healthy individuals. The three groups presented a colonization of 27% of the nostrils and a high prevalence of the superantigen SEA was found. The highest prevalence of *S. aureus* SEA + colonization was found in patients with recurrence or exacerbation of the disease [14].

The results describing the exacerbation of MS by bacterial superantigens, however, are contradictory. França et al. [3] demonstrated that prior infection with *S. aureus TSST-1* + reduced symptoms and consequently the inflammation of the central nervous system in mice with EAE. Similar results were described by Kumar et al.[39], in which mice infected with *S. aureus* in the subclinical phase of EAE showed a protective effect on clinical signs of the disease, including reduction of the central nervous system inflammatory infiltrate and demyelination of the optic nerve. The authors attributed the protective effect to the secretion of an extracellular protein (EAP) produced by *S. aureus* [40, 39].

In addition to participating in autoimmune pathologies, *S. aureus* has also been described as the most common bacteria in cases of septic arthritis [41]. The immunopathogenesis of septic arthritis (SA) is described as a joint disease that can occur from an infection elsewhere in the body, and bacteremia and sepsis are the most common [42]. This bacterium has many virulence factors inhibiting the immune response of the host, for example, collagen binding proteins, *clumping* factor A and B, extracellular adhesion matrix, enzymes, toxins, and superantigens [43, 44, 45]. Additionally, there are reports that immunocompromised patients are more susceptible to developing these types of disease; for example, elderly people, people with diabetes, people with rheumatoid arthritis, joint prosthesis users, intraarticular corticosteroid users, continuous users of central or peripheral venous catheters and people with skin infections [46, 47]. The development and pathogenic mechanisms of septic arthritis in humans are still unknown, but the frequent use of experimental models in research has substantially contributed to new findings [41].

## ARTHRITIS EXPERIMENTAL MODELS

Several animal species spontaneously develop arthritis caused by *S. aureus* and could thus be used as experimental models. Intravenous inoculation of *S. aureus* in mice has been the preferred route for development of the disease. This route allows the bacteria to adapt to the environment inside the host, to survive the serum microbicide components, and finally, to spread to the synovial tissue and penetrate several structures until it reaches the articular cavity [48].

*S. aureus* LS-1 produces TSST-1 and this characteristic has been used to initiate septic arthritis when administered intravenously in mice [49]. The contribution of TSST-1 has been the suggested reason that producers of this toxin increase the severity of arthritis, when compared to strains that do not [50]. TSST-1 also accelerates the collagen-induced arthritis in DBA mice [51].

One characteristic of septic arthritis is the exacerbated inflammatory immune response in the infection region, resulting in cartilage destruction and bone erosion [48]. Infection by *S. aureus* is accompanied by recruitment of polymorphonuclear cells, activated macrophages, and T cell infiltrate [52]. The involvement of pro-inflammatory cytokines has also been reported. This bacterium can induce production of cytokines, such as TNF-$\alpha$, IFN-$\gamma$, IL-1, IL-2 e IL-6 [53, 54].

The effect of T cells in this disease is clearly defined, and the contribution of each cell type is also discussed, for example, the effect of IL-17. IL-17 is produced by Th17 and also by several other T cells of innate immunity [54], both in humans and in rheumatoid arthritis experimental models [55, 57], but its role in septic arthritis is unknown. Recently, Colavite-Machado et al. [57] demonstrated the arthritogenic effect of IL-17 in experimental models. They found high levels of this cytokine in spleen cell cultures of mice infected with *S. aureus* (ATCC 19095) positive enterotoxin C when compared to uninfected mice. The use of experimental models for arthritis development has demonstrated the involvement of many virulence factors, as well as the participation of immune cells in the pathogenesis of septic arthritis. The mechanisms by which bacterial virulence factors interact with its host, however, still require further investigation. More information is needed for the development of vaccines or new combinations of therapeutic drugs for passive immunization and the use of antibiotics to minimize the risk and consequences of an infectious disease. In this case, the use of experimental models to describe disease development and new treatment strategies is crucial for further research.

## REFERENCES

[1] Vanderhaeghen, W; Hermans, K; Haesebrouck, F; Butaye, P. Methicillin-resistant *Staphylococcus aureus* (MRSA) in food production animals. *Epidemiol Infect.*, 2010, 138(5),606-25. doi: 10.1017/S0950268809991567.

[2] Wertheim, HF; Melles, DC; Vos, MC; van Leeuwen, W; van Belkum, A; Verbrugh, HA; Nouwen, JL. The role of nasal carriage in *Staphylococcus aureus* infections. *Lancet Infect Dis.*, 2005,5(12), 751-62.

[3] França, TG; Chiuso-Minicucci, F; Zorzella-Pezavento, SF; Ishikawa, LL; da Rosa, LC; Colavite, PM; Marques, C; Ikoma, MR; da Cunha, M de L; Sartori, A. Previous infection with *Staphylococcus aureus* strains attenuated experimental encephalomyelitis. *BMC Neurosci.*, 2014, 9, 15-8. doi: 10.1186/1471-2202-15-8.

[4] Larkin, EA; Carman, RJ; Krakauer, T; Stiles, BG. *Staphylococcus aureus*: the toxic presence of a pathogen extraordinaire. *Curr Med Chem.*, 2009,16(30), 4003-19.

[5] Fluit AC. Livestock-associated *Staphylococcus aureus*. *Clin Microbiol Infect.*, 2012,18(8), 735-44. doi: 10.1111/j.1469-0691.2012.03846.x.

[6] Lowy FD. *Staphylococcus aureus* infections. *N Engl J Med.*, 1998, 20, 339(8), 520-32.

[7] Spaulding, AR; Salgado-Pabón, W; Kohler, PL; Horswill, AR; Leung, DY; Schlievert, PM. Staphylococcal and streptococcal superantigen exotoxins. *Clin Microbiol Rev.*, 2013, 26(3), 422-47. doi: 10.1128/CMR.00104-12.

[8] Li, Z; Peres, AG; Damian, AC; Madrenas, J. Immunomodulation and Disease Tolerance to *Staphylococcus aureus*. *Pathogens.*, 2015, 13, 4(4), 793-815. doi: 10.3390/pathogens4040793.

[9] Murdoch, C; Finn, A. Chemokine receptors and their role in inflammation and infectious diseases. *Blood.*, 2000, 15, 95(10):3032-43.

[10] Montoya, M; Gouaux, E. Beta-barrel membrane protein folding and structure viewed through the lens of alpha-hemolysin. *Biochim Biophys Acta.*, 2003, 10, 1609(1), 19-27.

[11] Palmqvist, N; Foster, T; Tarkowski, A; Josefsson, E. Protein A is a virulence factor in *Staphylococcus aureus* arthritis and septic death. *Microb Pathog.*, 2002, 33(5), 239-49.

[12] Rooijakkers, SH; Ruyken, M; Roos, A; Daha, MR; Presanis, JS; Sim, RB; van Wamel, WJ; van Kessel, KP; van Strijp, JA. Immune evasion by staphylococcal complement inhibitor that acts on C3 convertases. *Nat Immunol.*, 2005, 6(9), 920-7.

[13] Lina, G; Bohach, GA; Nair, SP; Hiramatsu, K; Jouvin-Marche, E; Mariuzza, R. International Nomenclature Committee for Staphylococcal Superantigens. Standard nomenclature for the superantigens expressed by *Staphylococcus. J Infect Dis.*, 2004, 15, 189(12), 2334-6.

[14] Mulvey, MR; Doupe, M; Prout, M; Leong, C; Hizon, R; Grossberndt, A; Klowak, M; Gupta, A; Melanson, M; Gomori, A; Esfahani, F; Klassen, L; Frost, EE; Namaka, M. *Staphylococcus aureus* harbouring Enterotoxin A as a possible risk factor for multiple sclerosis exacerbations. *Mult Scler.*, 2011, 17(4), 397-403. doi: 10.1177/1352458510391343.

[15] Xu, SX; McCormick, JK. Staphylococcal superantigens in colonization and disease. *Front Cell Infect Microbiol.*, 2012, 17, 2:52. doi: 10.3389/fcimb.2012.00052.

[16] Foster TJ. Immune evasion by staphylococci. *Nat Rev Microbiol.*, 2005, 3(12), 948-58.

[17] Ortega, E; Abriouel, H; Lucas, R; Gálvez A. Multiple roles of Staphylococcus *aureus* enterotoxins: pathogenicity, superantigenic activity, and correlation to antibiotic resistance. *Toxins* (Basel), 2010, 2(8), 2117-31. doi: 10.3390/toxins2082117.

[18] Mollick, JA; Cook, RG; Rich, RR. Class II MHC molecules are specific receptors for staphylococcus enterotoxin A. *Science.*, 1989, 19, 244(4906), 817-20.

[19] Pontzer, CH; Russell, JK; Johnson, HM. Structural basis for differential binding of staphylococcal enterotoxin A and toxic shock syndrome toxin 1 to class II major histocompatibility molecules. *Proc Natl Acad Sci U S A.*, 1991, 1, 88(1), 125-8.

[20] Adorini L. Immunotherapeutic approaches in multiple sclerosis. *J Neurol Sci.* 2004, 15, 223(1), 13-24.

[21] Ursaciuc, C; Surcel, M; Ciotaru, D; Dobre, M; Pirvu, IR; Munteanu, AN; Alecu, M; Huică,R.Regulatory T cells and TH1/TH2 cytokines as immunodiagnosis keys in systemic autoimmune diseases. *Roum Arch Microbiol Immunol.*, 2010, 69(2), 79-84.

[22] Cosmi, L; Maggi, L; Santarlasci, V; Liotta, F; Annunziato, F. T helper cells plasticity in inflammation. *Cytometry A.*, 2014, 85(1), 36-42. doi: 10.1002/cyto.a.22348.

[23] Brocke, S; Gaur, A; Piercy, C; Gautam, A; Gijbels, K; Fathman, CG; Steinman, L. Induction of relapsing paralysis in experimental autoimmune encephalomyelitis by bacterial superantigen. *Nature.*, 1993, 14, 365(6447), 642-4.

[24] Mehrabi, F; Asgari, A. Resistant Strains of Enterotoxigenic *Staphylococcus aureus*; Unknown Risk for Multiple Sclerosis Exacerbation. *Iran Red Crescent Med J.*, 2015, 1, 17(9), e12596. doi: 10.5812/ircmj.12596.

[25] Swaminathan, S; Furey, W; Pletcher, J; Sax, M. Crystal structure of staphylococcal enterotoxin B, a superantigen. *Nature.*, 1992, 29, 359(6398), 801-6.

[26] Mantis NJ. Vaccines against the category B toxins: Staphylococcal enterotoxin B, epsilon toxin and ricin. *Adv Drug Deliv Rev.*, 2005, 17, 57(9), 1424-39.

[27] Argudín, MÁ; Mendoza, MC; Rodicio, MR. Food poisoning and *Staphylococcus aureus* enterotoxins. *Toxins (Basel).*, 2010, 2 (7), 1751-73. doi: 10.3390/toxins2071751.

[28] Teresa Krakauer and Bradley G Stiles. The staphylococcal enterotoxin (SE) family SEB and siblings. *Virulence.*, 2013, 4(8), 759–773. doi: 10.4161/viru.23905.

[29] Laouini, D; Kawamoto, S; Yalcindag, A; Bryce, P; Mizoguchi, E; Oettgen, H; Geha, RS. Epicutaneous sensitization with superantigen induces allergic skin inflammation. *J Allergy Clin Immunol.*, 2003, 112(5), 981-7.

[30] Li, J; Yang, J; Lu, YW; Wu, S; Wang, MR; Zhu, JM. Possible Role of Staphylococcal Enterotoxin B in the Pathogenesis of Autoimmune Diseases. *Viral Immunol.*, 2015, 28(7), 354-9. doi: 10.1089/vim.2015.0017.

[31] Schiffenbauer, J; Johnson, HM; Butfiloski, EJ; Wegrzyn, L; Soos, JM. Staphylococcal enterotoxins can reactivate experimental allergic encephalomyelitis. *Proc Natl Acad Sci U S A.*, 1993, 15, 90(18), 8543-6.

[32] Racke, MK; Quigley, L; Cannella, B; Raine, CS; McFarlin, DE; Scott, DE. Superantigen modulation of experimental allergic encephalomyelitis: activation of anergy determines outcome. *J Immunol.*, 1994, 15, 152(4), 2051-9.

[33] Soos, JM; Schiffenbauer, J; Johnson, HM. Treatment of PL/J mice with the superantigen, staphylococcal enterotoxin B, prevents development of experimental allergic encephalomyelitis. *J Neuroimmunol.*, 1993, 43(1-2), 39-43.

[34] Chowdhary, VR; Tilahun, AY; Clark, CR; Grande, JP; Rajagopalan, G. Chronic exposure to staphylococcal superantigen elicits a systemic inflammatory disease mimicking lupus. *J Immunol.*, 2012, 15, 189(4), 2054-62. doi: 10.4049/jimmunol.1201097.
[35] Kim, C; Siminovitch, KA; Ochi, A.Reduction of lupus nephritis in MRL/lpr mice by a bacterial superantigen treatment. *J Exp Med.*, 1991, 1, 174(6), 1431-7.
[36] Origuchi, T; Eguchi, K; Kawabe, Y; Yamashita, I; Mizokami, A; Ida, H; Nagataki, S.Increased levels of serum IgM antibody to staphylococcal enterotoxin B in patients with rheumatoid arthritis. *Ann Rheum Dis.*, 1995, 54(9), 713-20.
[37] Omata, S; Sasaki, T; Kakimoto, K; Yamashita, U. Staphylococcal enterotoxin B induces arthritis in female DBA/1 mice but fails to induce activation of type II collagen-reactive lymphocytes. *Cell Immunol.*, 1997, 1, 179(2), 138-45.
[38] Stinissen, P; Vandevyver, C; Raus, J; Zhang, J. Superantigen reactivity of gamma delta T cell clones isolated from patients with multiple sclerosis and controls. *Cell Immunol.*, 1995, 166(2), 227-35.
[39] Kumar, P; Kretzschmar, B; Herold, S; Nau, R; Kreutzfeldt, M; Schütze, S; Bähr, M; Hein, K. Beneficial effect of chronic *Staphylococcus aureus* infection in a model of multiple sclerosis is mediated through the secretion of extracellular adherence protein. *J Neuroinflammation.*, 2015, 3, 12, 22. doi: 10.1186/s12974-015-0241-8.
[40] Xie, C; Alcaide, P; Geisbrecht, BV; Schneider, D; Herrmann, M; Preissner, KT; Luscinskas, FW; Chavakis, T. Suppression of experimental autoimmune encephalomyelitis by extracellular adherence protein of *Staphylococcus aureus*. *J Exp Med.*, 2006, 17, 203(4), 985-94.
[41] Tarkowski A. Infection and musculoskeletal conditions: Infectious arthritis. *Best Pract Res Clin Rheumatol.*, 2006, 20(6), 1029-44.
[42] Edwards, AM; Massey, RC. Invasion of human cells by a bacterial pathogen. *J Vis Exp.*, 2011, 21, (49), pii, 2693. doi: 10.3791/2693.
[43] Switalski, LM; Patti, JM; Butcher, W; Gristina, AG; Speziale, P; Höök, M. A collagen receptor on *Staphylococcus aureus* strains isolated from patients with septic arthritis mediates adhesion to cartilage. *Mol Microbiol.*, 1993, 7(1), 99-107.

[44] Josefsson, E; Hartford, O; O'Brien, L; Patti, JM; Foster, T. Protection against experimental *Staphylococcus aureus* arthritis by vaccination with clumping factor A, novel virulence determinant. *J Infect Dis.*, 2001, 184(12), 1572-80.

[45] Ferry, T; Perpoint, T; Vandenesch, F; Etienne, J. Virulence determinants in *Staphylococcus aureus* and their involvement in clinical syndromes. *Curr Infect Dis Rep.*, 2005, 7(6), 420-8.

[46] Bonnal, C; Birgand, G; Lolom, I; Diamantis, S; Dumortier, C; L'Heriteau, F; Armand-Lefevre, L; Lucet, JC. *Staphylococcus aureus* healthcare associated bacterenia: An indicator of catheter related infections. *Med Mal Infect.*, 2015, 45(3), 84-8. doi: 10.1016/j.medmal.2015.01.002.

[47] Wang, DA; Tambyah, PA. Septic arthritis in immunocompetent and immunosuppressed hosts. *Best Pract Res Clin Rheumatol.*, 2015, 29(2), 275-89. doi: 10.1016/j.berh.2015.05.008.

[48] Colavite, PM; Ishikawa, LL; Zorzella-Pezavento, SF; de Oliveira, LR; França, TG; da Rosa, LC; Chiuso-Minicucci, F; Vieira, AE; Francisconi, CF; da Cunha, MLRS;Garlet,GP; Sartori,A.Cloxacillin control of experimental arthritis induced by SEC+ *Staphylococcus aureus* is associated with down modulation of local and systemic cytokines. *Cell Microbiol.*, 2015, 23. doi: 10.1111/cmi.12563.

[49] Sakiniene, E; Tarkowski, A. Low molecular weight heparin aggravates infectious arthritis triggered by *Staphylococcus aureus*. *J Orthop Res.*, 2002, 20(2), 198-203.

[50] Abdelnour, A; Bremell, T; Tarkowski, A. Toxic shock syndrome toxin 1 contributes to the arthritogenicity of *Staphylococcus aureus*. *J Infect Dis.*, 1994, 170(1), 94-9.

[51] Kageyama, Y; Koide, Y; Nagata, T; Uchijima, M; Yoshida, A; Arai, T; Miura, T; Miyamoto, C; Nagano, A. Toxic shock syndrome toxin-1 accelerated collagen-induced arthritis in mice. *J Autoimmun.*, 2001, 16(2), 125-31.

[52] Bremell, T; Abdelnour, A; Tarkowski, A. Histopathological and serological progression of experimental *Staphylococcus aureus* arthritis. *Infect Immun.*, 1992, 60(7), 2976-85.

[53] Saidenberg-Kermanac'h, N; Corrado, A; Lemeiter, D; deVernejoul, MC; Boissier MC; Cohen-Solal, ME. TNF alpha antibodies and osteoprotegerin decrease systemic bone loss associated with inflammation throughdistinct mechanisms in collagen-induced arthritis. *Bone.*, 2004, 35(5), 1200-7.

[54] Satorres, SE; Alcaráz, LE; Cargnelutti, E; Di Genaro, MS. IFN gamma plays a detrimental role in murine defense against nasal colonization of *Staphylococcus aureus. Immunol Lett.*, 2009, 27, 123(2), 185-8. doi: 10.1016/j.imlet.2009.03.003.

[55] Kim, JS; Jordan, MS. Diversity of IL-17-producing T lymphocytes. *Cell Mol Life Sci.*, 2013, 70(13), 2271-90. doi: 10.1007/s00018-012-1163-6.

[56] Nakae, S; Nambu, A; Sudo, K; Iwakura, Y. Suppression of immune induction of collagen-induced arthritis in IL-17-deficient mice. *J Immunol.*, 2003, 1, 171(11), 6173-7.

[57] Colavite-Machado, PM; Ishikawa, LL; França, TG; Zorzella-Pezavento, SF; da Rosa, LC; Chiuso-Minicucci, F; Cunha, MLRS; Garlet, GP; Sartori, A. Differential arthritogenicity of *Staphylococcus aureus* strains isolated from biological samples. *BMC Infect Dis.*, 2013, 30, 13, 400. doi: 10.1186/1471-2334-13-400.

# ABOUT THE EDITOR

**Maria de Lourdes Ribeiro de Souza da Cunha**, MD in Science and Technology of the Food (1992), PhD in Tropical Diseases (1998); is biologist with main research interests in Microbiology, focusing on Bacteriology, acting on the following subjects: *Staphylococcus aureus*, Coagulase-Negative Staphylococci (CoNS), epidemiology, virulence factors, biofilms, enterotoxins and antimicrobial resistance.

She is professor and researcher at the Department of Microbiology and Immunology of the Bioscience Institute, São Paulo State University (UNESP), Botucatu, SP, Brazil; Scholarship in Research Productivity of the National Council for Scientific and Technological Development (CNPq), an agency linked to the Ministry of Science and Tecnology (MCT), dedicated to the promotion of scientific and technological research and to the formation of human resources for research in the Brazil. Professor and mentor master's, doctoral and postdoctoral studies at the graduate program in Tropical Diseases, Faculty of Medicine of Botucatu and the Post-graduation in General Biology and Applied, Biosciences Institute, UNESP, Botucatu, SP, Brazil. She is involved in research projects as a scientific reference in *Staphylococcus* supported for the São Paulo Research Foundation – FAPESP – public foundation with the mission to foster research and the scientific and technological development of the State of São Paulo, Brazil. She is the author of more than 80 papers in international peer reviewed journals and books, and referee for about 20 journals.

# INDEX

## #

β chain, 117

## A

a catheter, 12, 88
abscesses, 12, 90
accurate, xii, 12, 66, 69, 70
*Acinetobacter baumannii*, 10
adaptability, xi, 27, 50
Alpha-toxin, 5
aminoglycosides, 8
anergy, 5, 118, 124
animals, xi, 4, 36, 37, 38, 39, 40, 41, 42, 44, 45, 47, 49, 50, 53, 54, 55, 56, 58, 60, 64, 88, 116, 122
antibiotic resistance, x, 3, 4, 8, 57, 76, 78, 123
antigen presenting cells, 115, 117
antigen receptors, 117
antimicrobial susceptibility testing, 8, 69, 78, 80
arthritis, 116, 119, 120, 121, 122, 125, 126, 127
autoimmune diseases, xii, 116, 117, 118, 119, 123
automation, 66, 70
axillae, 14

## B

beef, 39
beta-lactams, 2, 7, 8, 27, 31
beta-toxin, 6, 16
biochemical tests, 70, 74
biofilm, 5, 6, 13, 16, 52, 57, 74, 75, 104, 106, 108, 109, 114
bloodstream infection, xii, 11, 12, 13, 52, 65, 66, 67, 69, 72, 73, 74, 75, 78, 84, 87, 88, 90, 93
bone erosion, 121
bones, 12
breastfeeding, 90, 92
burn, x, 1, 2, 3, 4, 7, 10, 11, 12, 13, 14, 17, 18, 19, 20, 22, 23, 57

## C

capsule, 5
carriers, 29, 30, 33, 51, 53, 90, 92, 104, 109, 113
cartilage, 121, 125
catalase-positive, 4
catheters, x, 2, 5, 13, 27, 68, 86, 92, 104, 106, 120
cattle, xi, 36, 38, 40, 41, 45, 64
cefazolin, 110
Ceftaroline, 14, 22
Ceftobiprole, 8, 14, 22

cephalosporins, 13, 14
chemotaxis, 115, 116
chicken, xi, 39, 40, 45
chloramphenicol, 8
chlorexidine, 14
chronic wounds, 26, 29
clindamycin, 2, 8, 52, 54, 55
clinical microbiology laboratory, 69
clones, x, 2, 3, 8, 9, 10, 15, 18, 27, 32, 49, 56, 57, 58, 59, 62, 92, 125
coagulase, ix, 4, 12, 17, 63, 65, 67, 68, 70, 75, 76, 77, 79, 84, 87, 88, 97, 104, 105, 112, 117, 129
community-associated methicillin-resistant *S. aureus* (CA-MRSA), x, 2, 3, 6, 7, 8, 10, 25, 26, 27, 28, 30, 31, 36, 37, 38, 41, 50, 51, 53, 55, 56, 57, 58
control, 1, 2, 3, 8, 9, 10, 14, 17, 19, 20, 22, 26, 30, 32, 33, 41, 45, 54, 55, 59, 67, 73, 83, 85, 89, 91, 92, 94, 95, 96, 98, 99, 100, 101, 109, 126
conventional antigens, 117
copper, 58
cross-contamination, 3
cross-transmission, 14, 15, 85
cytokine, 72, 77, 121
cytolytic, 5, 6, 16
cytolytic toxins, 5, 16

## D

daptomycin, 8, 13, 22, 111
daycare, 54
diabetes, xi, 30, 105, 107, 108, 120
diagnosis, xi, 11, 12, 20, 65, 69, 71, 76, 77, 78, 81, 84, 95
dissemination, x, xi, 3, 4, 9, 27, 36, 39, 41, 50, 89, 92
dogs, 55, 59
drug, 22, 26, 28, 30, 33, 56, 63, 95, 110, 124

## E

early, 55, 65, 69, 75, 77, 78, 84, 87, 93, 96, 118
elderly, xi, 26, 29, 32, 51, 120
encephalitis, 118, 120
environment, x, 39, 40, 44, 51, 56, 69, 85, 86, 91, 92, 107, 121
epidemiology, ix, x, 1, 2, 3, 4, 9, 17, 19, 20, 22, 31, 32, 33, 35, 36, 37, 38, 40, 41, 42, 43, 49, 50, 59, 64, 67, 72, 74, 76, 94, 97, 99, 104, 113, 129
evasion, 5, 16, 42, 115, 116, 123
exfoliative toxins, 5, 51, 106
extracellular enzymes, 5
extracellular factors, 4
extrinsic, 86

## F

facultative anaerobic, 4
farmers, 36, 38, 53
fever, 10, 12, 55, 66, 87, 108, 119
food, xi, 37, 39, 40, 42, 44, 45, 84, 118, 122, 124, 129
fusidic acid, 58

## G

gram staining, 70
gram-negative bacilli, 10, 67
gram-positive bacteria, 4
gram-positive cocci, 67, 70, 80, 88, 104, 105

## H

hand hygiene, 14, 22, 30, 93
histocompatibility molecules, 117, 123
HIV/AIDS patients, 29
homeostasis, 117
hospital-acquired infections, 4, 36

# Index

hospitalization, x, xii, 1, 26, 27, 29, 86, 90, 91, 98, 104, 105, 111
host immune response, 5, 107
host tissues, 5
household, 53
housekeeping genes, 9

## I

identification, x, xi, 4, 9, 16, 27, 65, 69, 70, 71, 74, 75, 77, 78, 79, 80, 81, 97, 107, 112
immobile, 4
immunocompromised, 4, 27, 37, 68, 120
incidence, 12, 20, 28, 33, 41, 65, 66, 72, 87, 91, 93, 95, 98, 100
infection, x, xi, xii, 1, 2, 4, 5, 6, 8, 9, 10, 11, 12, 14, 15, 18, 19, 20, 22, 27, 29, 30, 32, 38, 39, 40, 41, 42, 44, 45, 47, 51, 52, 53, 54, 55, 56, 57, 62, 63, 64, 66, 67, 74, 83, 84, 85, 86, 87, 88, 89, 90, 91, 92, 93, 94, 97, 98, 99, 100, 101, 104, 105, 106, 107, 108, 109, 110, 113, 114, 120, 121, 122, 125
infection control strategies, 4, 93
insulin, 26, 30
intermittent, 109
intrinsic, 86
invasive devices, 26, 29, 66
invasive diseases, 58
ionization, 70, 80, 108, 112
irritability, 87
isolation, 14, 15, 22, 40, 45, 51, 52, 53, 54, 69, 75, 77, 85

## J

joints, 12, 119

## K

kidney, 110, 111, 113, 114, 119

## L

late, 77, 84, 87, 88, 95, 98
lesions, 26, 105
linezolid, 8, 13, 21, 76, 111, 114
lipases, 5, 105
livestock-associated, xi, 37, 42, 43, 44, 45, 46, 49, 50, 54, 64, 122
lock therapy, 13
long-term care facilities, xi, 26, 29, 90
lupus, 116, 118, 119, 125
lymphocytes, 5, 6, 29, 117, 125, 127

## M

macrolides, 8, 53
mass spectrometry, 70, 80, 112
mastitis, 36, 39, 52, 61, 90
metabolism, 66, 70, 107
methicillin, ix, 1, 2, 7, 15, 16, 17, 18, 19, 21, 22, 23, 26, 27, 30, 31, 32, 33, 35, 36, 38, 42, 43, 44, 45, 46, 47, 50, 54, 55, 58, 59, 60, 61, 62, 63, 64, 74, 75, 76, 81, 84, 89, 93, 94, 97, 98, 99, 100, 101, 104, 106, 110, 111, 112, 116, 122
microbiota, 66, 68, 85, 86, 88
microdilution, 70
milk products, 39
misidentification, 71
molecular biology, 66, 71
molecular tools, xi, 50
mortality, xi, xii, 2, 8, 12, 27, 30, 36, 37, 56, 58, 64, 65, 66, 67, 69, 72, 78, 84, 86, 88, 90, 95, 103, 105, 108, 111
mucous membranes, 4, 5, 28, 68, 116
multilocus sequence typing, 9, 57
multiple antibiotic resistance, 3
multiple sclerosis, 116, 117, 118, 120, 123, 125
mupirocin, 30, 64, 104, 109, 113
myelin, 116, 117, 118

## N

nasal and pharyngeal colonization, 3
necrosis, 5, 6, 10
necrotizing pneumonia, 6, 52
needles, 30, 68
newborn, 52, 60, 85, 86, 94, 95, 96
nosocomial, x, xi, xii, 2, 4, 8, 9, 20, 21, 26, 27, 37, 41, 42, 43, 66, 67, 72, 73, 74, 76, 78, 84, 88, 91, 92, 93, 94, 95, 96, 97, 98, 100, 112

## O

opportunistic microorganisms, 68
opsonization, 5
outbreaks, 9, 30, 83, 85, 91, 99
outcome, 21, 72, 74, 94, 105, 107, 108, 112, 113, 124

## P

penicillin-binding protein, 3, 7
peptides, 6, 16, 117
perineum, 14
peritoneal dialysis, xii, 68, 103, 111, 112, 113, 114
peritoneal membrane, 103, 105
peritonitis, xii, 68, 103, 105, 106, 107, 108, 109, 110, 111, 112, 113, 114
phenol-soluble modulin, 5, 6, 52
phenotypic methods, 70, 71, 75
photometry, 70
pig, 38, 46, 60, 63
poor feeding, 87
poultry, 38, 39, 40, 44, 56
prematurity, 83, 84, 86, 88, 91
pressure ulcers, 52
prevention, ix, 11, 12, 15, 17, 20, 22, 30, 32, 45, 73, 83, 85, 92, 93, 94, 103, 105, 110
prognosis, xi, xii, 69, 104, 105
proteases, 5, 118
protein A, 5, 9, 16, 18, 42, 122
*Pseudomonas aeruginosa*, 10

pulsed-field gel electrophoresis, 9, 18
purulent, 54

## Q

quinolones, 8
quinupristin/dalfopristin, 8, 111

## R

raw milk, 39
recurrence, xii, 105, 110, 117, 120
relapse, 110, 117, 120
retail meat products, 39
rheumatoid arthritis, 118, 119, 120, 121, 125
rifampicin, 110, 111
risk factors, 2, 4, 12, 19, 26, 27, 29, 38, 54, 83, 86, 88, 91, 104

## S

sepsis, xi, 10, 12, 15, 18, 25, 27, 31, 36, 67, 68, 69, 70, 72, 73, 76, 77, 78, 84, 86, 87, 88, 90, 92, 93, 94, 95, 96, 98, 116, 120
septic shock, 69, 77, 78
silver sulfadiazine, 11
skin, xi, 3, 4, 6, 7, 8, 10, 11, 12, 13, 14, 15, 21, 25, 27, 28, 29, 30, 43, 51, 52, 53, 60, 62, 68, 77, 85, 86, 88, 90, 93, 116, 118, 120, 124
soft tissue, 7, 8, 10, 14, 21, 22, 25, 27, 41, 51, 90
*spa* typing, 9, 52, 57
staff, 51, 105
staphylococcal chromosome cassette *mec*, 3
staphylococcal enterotoxin-like, 5
staphylococcal enterotoxins, 5, 51, 106, 124
strains, x, xi, 2, 3, 4, 6, 7, 8, 27, 28, 30, 36, 37, 38, 39, 40, 41, 44, 45, 47, 49, 50, 51, 52, 53, 54, 55, 56, 57, 58, 63, 64, 80, 89, 90, 92, 93, 106, 107, 108, 116, 121, 122, 124, 125, 127
sulfamethoxazole-trimethoprim, 8

superantigens, xii, 5, 16, 104, 105, 106, 115, 116, 117, 118, 120, 123
surfactant, 6, 14
surgical procedures, 12
surveillance, 2, 4, 12, 14, 15, 20, 42, 51, 54, 59, 66, 67, 72, 73, 74, 79, 91, 92, 94, 95, 98, 99, 100
survival, 30, 40, 69, 77, 78, 86, 92, 100
systemic activation, 118

## T

T cells, 115, 117, 118, 121, 123
tetracycline, 8, 51, 52, 53, 55
tigecycline, 8, 14
toxic shock syndrome toxin 1, 5, 106, 123, 126
toxins, 5, 15, 56, 66, 87, 104, 105, 106, 107, 108, 112, 115, 116, 120, 123, 124

treatment, 1, iii, xi, xii, 8, 17, 18, 21, 22, 40, 51, 66, 69, 77, 78, 84, 85, 93, 103, 104, 106, 108, 110, 113, 114, 121, 124, 125

## V

Vancomycin, 2, 8, 13, 14, 17, 21, 22, 32, 55, 107, 108, 110
ventilator-associated pneumonia, 11, 12, 19, 52, 78
veterinarians, 36, 38, 40, 46, 53, 59, 63
virulence, x, 2, 3, 4, 5, 6, 8, 15, 16, 26, 30, 31, 35, 36, 42, 49, 50, 51, 52, 56, 57, 58, 59, 63, 64, 75, 86, 104, 105, 106, 107, 112, 120, 121, 122, 124, 126, 129

## W

wound, 1, 3, 10, 11, 12, 13, 18, 19, 51, 52, 53, 57, 90

SOUTHERN REGIONAL TECHNICAL COLLEGE GEORGIA